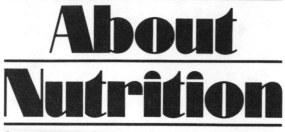

About
Nutrition

Seventh-day Adventist Dietetic Association

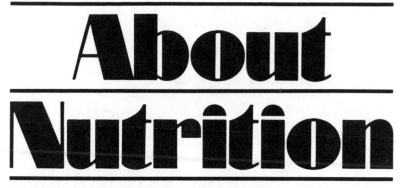

About Nutrition

Seventh-day Adventist Dietetic Association

Authors
Alice G. Marsh, Sc.D., R.D.
Rose G. Stoia, Ed.D., R.D.
Dorothy Christensen, M.S., R.D.
Sylvia M. Fagal, M.S., R.D.

Second Revised Edition

REVIEW AND HERALD PUBLISHING ASSOCIATION
Washington, DC 20039-0555
Hagerstown, MD 21740

Copyright © 1986 by
Review and Herald Publishing Association

This book was
Edited by Richard W. Coffen
Designed by Richard Steadham
Cover photo by David B. Sherwin
Type set: 10/11 Century School Book

PRINTED IN U.S.A.

Library of Congress Cataloging in Publication Data

Main entry under title:

About Nutrition.

 Bibliography: p. 155
 Includes index.
 1. Vegetarianism. 2. Nutrition. I. Marsh, Alice G.
II. Seventh-day Adventist Dietetic Association.
TX392.A422 1986 613.2 85-18441
ISBN 0-8280-0238-X

Table of Contents

7/Nutrition Information

11/Preface

13/For Your Information

SECTION I

NUGGETS OF KNOWLEDGE ON NUTRIENTS

16/Four Food Groups Fit
29/Body's Big Business
34/The Fire of Life
50/In the Ashes
57/Everybody Loves a Vitamin

SECTION II

TAILORING ACCORDING TO NEED

70/Lifetime Nutrition
83/Engineered Curves
90/Teeth That Last
93/Reducing Health Risks

SECTION III

FOOD FUNDAMENTALS

100/Food Puzzle Applied
115/Chemist in the Kitchen
120/Artist at Work

SECTION IV

ON YOUR GUARD

132/Poison in the Pot
137/Current Quackery
142/Food Fads and Facts

APPENDIX

152/Recommended Daily Dietary Allowances
154/U.S. Dietary Goals
155/Bibliography
157/Index

Nutrition Information

Alford, Betty B., and Margaret L. Bogle. *Nutrition During the Life Cycle*. Englewood Cliffs, N.J.: Prentice-Hall, 1982.

Brody, Jane. *Jane Brody's Nutrition Book*. New York: Bantam Books, 1982.

Endres, Jeannette B., and Robert E. Rockwell. *Food, Nutrition, and the Young Child*. St. Louis: C. V. Mosby Company, 1980.

Fagal, Sylvia M. *Nutrition Helps*. Loma Linda, Calif.: Seventh-day Adventist Dietetics Association, n.d.

Goldbeck, Nikki, and David Goldbeck. *American Wholefoods Cuisine*. New York: New American Library, 1983.

Hafen, Brent Q. *Nutrition, Food, and Weight Control*. Expanded ed. Boston: Allyn and Bacon, 1981.

Heslin, Jo-Ann, Annette Natow, and Barbara Raven. *No-Nonsense Nutrition for Your Baby's First Year*. Boston: CBI Publishing Company, 1978.

Kart, Cary S., and Seamus P. Metress. *Nutrition, the Aged, and Society*. Englewood Cliffs, N.J.: Prentice-Hall, 1984.

Mayer, Jean. *A Diet for Living*. New York: David McKay Company, 1975.

McGill, Marion, and Orrea Pye. *The No-Nonsense Guide to Food and Nutrition*. New York: Butterick Publishing, 1978.

Notelowitz, Morris, and Marsha Ware. *Stand Tall! The Informed Woman's Guide to Preventing Osteoporosis*. Gainesville, Fla.: Triad Publishing Company, 1982.

Stare, Fredrick J., and Margaret McWilliams. *Nutrition for Good Health*. Fullerton, Calif.: Plycon Press, 1974.

White, Philip, and Nancy Selvey. *Let's Talk About Food*. Acton, Mass.: Publishing Sciences Group, 1974.

Acknowledgments

The authors continue to appreciate the work of those who aided in the planning and coordinating of the first version of *About Nutrition*—Darlene R. Schmitz, R.D.; Royalynn B. Case, M.S., R.D.; and Barbara J. Myers, M.S., R.D. The title, *About Nutrition,* was suggested by Clinton A. Wall, B.S., R.D., who also aided greatly in developing its philosophy and organization. The Seventh-day Adventist Dietetic Association publication committee in office during the initial writing of the book—Ruth Little Carey, Ph.D., R.D., chairperson; Kathleen K. Zolber, Ph.D., R.D.; Irma B. Vyhmeister, D.P.H., R.D.; and Ardis S. Beckner, M.S., R.D.—evaluated the material and gave excellent suggestions. A number of other skilled readers offered valued editorial refinement.

Recent officers of the Seventh-day Adventist Dietetic Association have encouraged the authors to continue in the revision of the book to keep it available for worldwide use as a text for students, a guide for homemakers, and a reference for food administrators.

Preface

Utilizing today's advances in science and nutrition research, the Seventh-day Adventist Dietetic Association presents this volume in its second revision. The book has four sections.

Section I sets the theme for the entire book, using the Four Food Groups as the basis for meeting daily nutritional needs. This section serves as a concise reference text in nutrition. The author of this section originated the food "puzzle" that serves as a simple guide to maintaining the excellent nutrition this book advocates throughout.

Section II presents guidelines for adjusting the Four Food Groups to meet the nutritional needs from childhood to old age. The authors also discuss nutrition management during common illnesses.

Section III guides those responsible for menu planning and food budgets to include the Four Food Groups wisely. It shows how to prepare food in the most appealing way, yet conserving the nutritional value.

Section IV helps the reader establish a sound program of nutrition by using familiar foods available in local markets. It also presents the dangers of fad diets with limited food selection.

The book advocates the lacto-ovo-vegetarian diet as adequate and advantageous within the framework of the Four Food Groups. In this diet, milk (lacto), eggs (ovo), and plant sources (vegetarian) in the form of fruits, vegetables, grains, and nuts provide all nutrients abundantly. The authors explain the advantages of a lacto-ovo-vegetarian diet during a century when heart and other degenerative diseases are major causes of disability and death.

The respective authors as listed on the title page of this second revision of *About Nutrition* have written the sections of the book in the order presented. Each author strongly advocates good nutrition obtained by way of an intelligent selection of good food. They concertedly recommend the convenient guide presented for use in daily food choice. Persons of all ages can be nourished in a way that promotes health and a zest for life and that avoids the pitfalls of fads, nutritional misinformation, and quackery, which lead to a waste of life and resources.

The 1980 Recommended Dietary Allowances of the Food and Nutrition Board of the National Research Council, National Academy of Sciences, have been used to verify the adequacy of the lacto-ovo-vegetarian diet. For a convenient dietary analysis reference, the reader should obtain Home and Garden Bulletin No. 72 from the United States Department of Agriculture, Superintendent of Documents, U.S. Government Printing Office, Washington, D.C. 20402, and/or for a more complete reference, *Nutritive Value of American Food in Common Units,* U.S. Department of Agriculture Handbook No. 456, same address.

As this second revised edition of *About Nutrition* goes to press the expected 10th edition of the Recommended Dietary Allowances by the Food and Nutrition Board of the National Research Council has not been released. Since *About Nutrition* bases good nutritional practices on proper food selection, small changes in recommended allowances will not affect this guide. The one possible exception is calcium intake for women. Based on available research and present knowledge, we give this recommendation on page 52.

For Your Information

This book, based on the lacto-ovo-vegetarian diet, presents a way of life that includes the use of all good food. Normal nutrition ensues only when the food adequately supplies all essential nutrients. Good health follows good nutrition. Poor health inevitably results from poor nutrition.

Normally, undernutrition will not happen when one chooses a daily diet from ordinary foods according to the pattern of the Four Food Groups. Neither will overnutrition cause toxicity. The puzzle is easily put together. Each day as the individual homemaker or the food service manager chooses from the four groups of food, he/she utilizes the metaphysics of the ages and the biochemistry of this century to feed each person. Each individual fed is most fortunate that he lives where food is available, when nutrition has become a well-understood science, and with someone who cares enough to provide food that nourishes the body for its best function and longest duration. The individual can with dexterity and confidence walk the tightrope of good nutrition—enough of all the good nutrients he needs but not too much to unbalance the perfect metabolic processes of the human body.

The nutrients discussed throughout the book come from good everyday food. Food comes from the field, garden, orchard, and dairy, or for most people from the various food markets. Each person feeding himself or others should consider it a privilege to learn the principles of good food preparation in order to preserve nutrients while he readies the food in the most acceptable form for life at its best.

With so many food and varieties of foods from which to choose, everyone should become a scientist to the extent that he knows how to utilize the sciences vital to life. He should become an artist to the extent that the science of living is also an art. Then the science and art of eating should take only their rightful place as a natural part of life, supporting the spiritual and intellectual facets that involve life in its highest sense of values.

Section I

Nuggets of Knowledge on Nutrients
16/Four Food Groups Fit
29/Body's Big Business
34/The Fire of Life
50/In the Ashes
57/Everybody Loves a Vitamin

Chapter 1

FOUR FOOD GROUPS FIT

The happiest discovery about nutrition is that good nutrition results from eating ordinary food. Readily available food is the source of good nutrition as nature's God intended. In contrast to a "pill or potion" generation of health seekers, this book does not outguess or try to outsmart nature. Nutrients depend upon balances that only food can provide—calcium balanced with phosphorus, vitamin A with vitamin E, vitamin C with calcium and certain of the amino acids of protein, to name a few. Food can provide these balances without deficiencies and without megadoses. The former can cause disease and death, and the latter can produce serious imbalances and even vitamin and mineral "poisoning."

The scientist and the nonscientist alike, to attain good nutrition and maintain good health, need a daily guide in choosing a diet from the abundance of food given by the provident Creator. Everyone bears the responsibility for food selection, preservation, preparation, and consumption, and it does not go away. Although the homemaker or the food service administrator assumes the greater share of the task, the individual consumer makes the final decision as to how much good nutrition, good art, good fun, and good living mix with the food he eats.

The attitudes associated with choosing daily food should not center entirely around the inquiry "What do I like?" but rather, "Which foods will give the best possible body function and upkeep as well as enjoyment for today?" The person who has learned to like good food discovers that the very foods he likes best fit into a plan assuring good nutrition.

Conveniently, good nutrition possesses a "least common denominator" known as the Four Food Groups, which resembles a simple preschool puzzle. Like all puzzles, they make sense when put together, but they do not go together unless each piece fits exactly into its place. One piece cannot replace another.

The Four Food Groups idea has succeeded as a guide for daily diet planning because it encompasses all foods that nature provides.

Besides this, the foods of most world cultures (except in areas where civilization exceeds food acquisition) fit into this basic plan. Thus the individual choosing his food can select any of the foods available to him—from all fruits and vegetables, from all cereals and breads, from all foods that contribute liberally to the body's need for protein, from all dairy products or their alternates. One survey revealed the abundance of foods fitting into the plan by discovering sixty-six varieties of fresh, fresh-frozen, and canned vegetables available year-round in one Midwestern small-town area. Although foods fit into but four groups, the selection in each group is amazingly abundant and variable.

Four servings each day from the first two groups and two servings each day from the second two groups constitute the daily minimum from the Four Food Groups.

Fruit and Vegetable Group .... 4 servings
    1 serving of which provides a good source of vitamin C
      (citrus fruit, tomatoes, or fresh raw vegetables)
    1 serving of which provides a good source of vitamin A
      (a very dark-green or deep yellow vegetable)
Cereal and Bread Group .... 4 servings
    Whole-grain or enriched; at least 2 servings whole-grain
Protein Group .... 2 servings
Milk Group .... 2 servings
    Low-fat or skim for adults

The Food Groups Make a Nutritional Puzzle Fit

Fruit and Vegetable Group

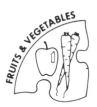

The fruit and vegetable group includes an almost endless variety of foods. Parents should introduce them to every child after early infancy so he may learn to accept various tastes. The body converts certain carotenes into vitamin A. One serving of cooked or raw

AN-2

17

carrots, broccoli, yellow squash or pumpkin, rutabaga, or any of the dark-green greens assures enough vitamin A.*

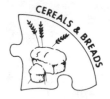

One certain cereal usually predominates in the diet of each distinct world culture. In countries composed of various old cultures, the citizens tend toward better nourishment when they have learned to like a variety of cereal grains served in many ways. The use of various cereal grains not only improves nutrition but also adds social interest to everyday eating. Cereal grains, depended upon as the primary dietary staple, are relatively inexpensive, available, and satisfying—a bland food that combines well with colorful and highly flavorful foods.

For the most part, select cereals and breads from whole grains. Whenever certain people who have some types of digestive problems are advised to use cereals and flours with the roughest outer hull milled off or else finely ground whole-grain flour, they should be certain all refined flour and cereal used are enriched. Probably a good rule for meal planning is be sure: *at least* half of the cereals and breads are made from whole grains.

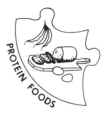

---

* Interestingly, a food may play a double role in the menu. For instance, sweet potatoes serve as both the starchy vegetable and the food with a high vitamin A value. A spinach quiche can serve as a protein-food serving and a vitamin A vegetable. Pizza provides a bread, a vegetable, and a good protein food. Most vegetable juices served as a beverage also abound in vitamin A. When you use a lesser green or yellow vegetable such as peas, green or wax beans, asparagus, or lima beans, which have less vitamin A value, select a dark-green or deep-yellow vegetable the next day.

This group of foods should supply most of the vitamin C for the day. A small serving of citrus fruit, a half cup of its juice, and a serving of freshly prepared cabbage are examples of excellent sources of this vitamin.

The protein food group includes the large variety of legumes (mature beans and peas), eggs and egg dishes, gluten (wheat protein), soy products (including tofu), and many tasty combinations. Whether produced at home or by food companies, these foods make excellent vegetable protein meat analogs.* Nuts and nut butters contribute some protein to the diet, but because with few exceptions nuts have more fat than any other nutrient, they are not major contributors of protein in a well-managed diet. In the nonvegetarian diet, lean meat, fish, and fowl fit into this group.

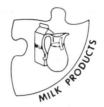

Milk and milk products contribute liberally to the protein needs of the body, but a separate milk group is needed to include certain nutrients the other food groups—including other protein foods—do not abundantly provide. The milk group assures calcium, riboflavin, vitamin B_{12}, and certain essential microminerals. Milk also efficiently provides proteins that supplement less effective proteins in other foods. Since milk is nutritionally efficient, include it in some form at each meal. You can serve whole milk, 2 percent fat milk, evaporated milk, skim milk (fluid, evaporated, or reconstituted dry), buttermilk, yogurt, or chocolate milk. Consider the latter a dessert and serve very moderately. Fortified soybean milk-type beverages adequately substitute for milk or may be used as a milk alternate. Cheese may contribute either as a milk-group serving or as a serving in the protein group.

---

* Meat analogs are made by General Foods Corporation, White Plains, New York; Loma Linda Foods, Riverside, California; Worthington Foods, Incorporated, Worthington, Ohio; and other companies.

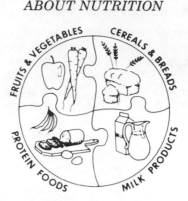

With the "least common denominator" (provided by the food groups) of good nutrition fitted together, everyone can add servings to make the daily diet fit his personal food requirements. To supply the needs of different ages and conditions, the Four Food Groups puzzle takes on a third dimension, according to the number of servings used. The individual who needs more food simply adds more servings from the food groups.

Adults

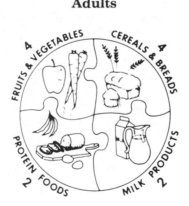

First of all, everyone needs each of the four pieces of the food groups stacked in the number indicated to represent the number of servings—4, 4, 2, 2 ("Food for Fitness: A Daily Food Guide," United States Department of Agriculture, Agricultural Research Service). This plan makes a good low-calorie diet for adults, since food choices from the Four Food Groups plan alone usually do not exceed 1,200 calories. If skim milk replaces whole milk, the plan constitutes a very satisfactory diet of approximately 1,000 calories. To add calories, a person should use more fruits, vegetables, and cereals, with limited amounts of "additions," (see page 23). Maintenance of proper weight for each individual determines the amount of additions to use.

Preschool Children

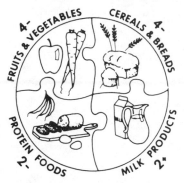

Little folks need the same foods as adults but in small or even tiny servings. Add an extra milk serving if it does not cause the young child to exclude foods of the other groups.

School-age Children

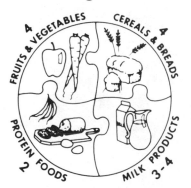

School-age youngsters may eat as much or more than their parents, plus extra milk. The amounts they require vary from child to child and for the same child from day to day. Providing enough of the proper food throughout the child's development is the parent's responsibility. The normal child who has learned to like good food usually eats the right amount for himself with a reasonable amount of "additions" (see page 23).

Teens

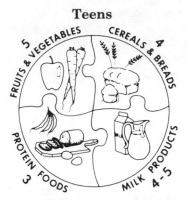

Teenagers and even preteens necessitate a third serving of protein food, an extra vitamin C food, and two or three extra servings of milk. Supply more energy foods, if needed, with others of the Four Food Groups foods, especially whole-grain cereal and bread selections. Select "additions" carefully to add energy food and to contribute to the abundance of nutrients demanded by the teen's growth and development. Teen treats and snacks should contribute protein, minerals, and vitamins, as well as calories.

Pregnancy

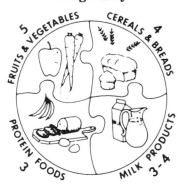

Pregnancy's extra nutritional requirements are met, first of all, by the woman's lifetime of good nutrition. Studies show that the years of good nutrition before conception as well as adequate nutrition during pregnancy provide the greatest assurance of proper development of the new life. Added to her normal diet, she needs one extra serving each of milk, a vitamin C food, and a protein food. As the demand of the developing child increases, the pregnant woman's nutritional puzzle requires servings as follows: 5, 4, 3, 3-4, respectively, of fruits and vegetables for vitamins A and C foods, cereals and breads, protein foods, and milk.

Lactation

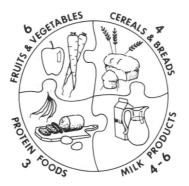

The lactating woman calls for further additions to the diet—from two to four extra servings of milk (this can be skim milk), two extra servings of a vitamin C food, and one extra protein food. Thus her food servings are a minimum of 6, 4, 3, 4-6, respectively, of fruits and vegetables, cereals and breads, protein foods, and milk.

Additions: A Few for Everyone—Very Little for Some

Common "additions" to the Four Food Groups are fats and sweets, which must be used sparingly. These additions include spreads, cooking fats, salad dressings, seed oils, olives, avocados, nuts, jellies and jams, syrups, honey, and sugars. When restricting your calories, use these additions sparingly—if at all—except for a minimum daily inclusion of approximately two teaspoons of a seed oil, such as corn oil. However, do not overlook the important addition of water. While adding zero calories, water is important to all functions of the body and vital to good nutrition. Choose it as a between-meal "snack" frequently during the day.

The good homemaker or the trained food service director provides each day the foods that complete the puzzle of the Four Food Groups and excludes no food from the pool of selections, but utilizes foods of all seasons, tapping nature's storehouse each day. Neither complicated meals nor a narrow selection need exist. Nutrition for every individual can be perfect.

Notice the following day's menu of typical foods selected from the Four Food Groups. The "additions" add appeal and satisfaction, enabling the individual to select sufficient total calories.

Breakfast
Orange slices
Rolled oats
Scrambled egg   Low-fat milk   50% whole-wheat toast

Dinner
Baked brown beans
Stuffed baked potato   Buttered cauliflower
Lettuce-and-tomato salad
Whole-wheat rolls   Soft-type margarine*
Ice cream with sweet wafers
Hot cereal drink made with low-fat milk

Supper or Lunch
Vegetable soup
Whole-wheat wafers
Peanut butter sandwiches   Low-fat milk   Stewed dried apricots

It is impractical and unnecessary to calculate the major nutrients in every day's meals. Utilization of the Four Food Groups as a guide in menu-making automatically assures their presence almost without exception. Choosing from a variety of foods will compensate for the possible exceptions.

For those who like to study figures, Table 1 calculates this menu for its calorie (kcal., or large calorie) content and for eight nutrients. It compares the totals of each with the recommended dietary allowances for men and for women suggested by the Food and Nutrition Board of the National Research Council "Recommended Dietary Allowances"—10th ed. [National Academy of Sciences, 1985]. It bases the recommendations on the average growth pattern of North Americans.

The choices from the Four Food Groups given in Table 1, pages 27, 28, furnish 1,156 calories. The "additions" on page twenty-eight increase the total calories to 1,973. Thus the menu basically supplies all nutritional requirements, except that most men require more food for sufficient calories (energy), and women may need more iron, which additional vegetables, fruits, and whole grains would provide.

---

* Liquid seed oil should be the first-stated ingredient.

ABOUT NUTRITION

The Four Food Groups form the basis of good food selection for the family. Individual family members can adapt to their specific dietary needs by availing themselves of more food selections and by making food "additions" wisely. Find the recommended dietary allowances for specific sex and age groups on pages 152, 153.

Much flexibility must be allowed for individuals to choose amounts of food. Some people are normally "easy keepers" by efficiently using nutrients. Other people are not. Some may need additional amounts of most nutrients, while others may need additional amounts of only one or two. Although the needs of individuals vary, people of the same age, sex, and within a moderate size range require surprisingly similar amounts of protein, minerals, and vitamins.

Individual teenage requirements vary the most. Nature intends some young persons to become larger than average in bone structure—some smaller. Some acquire their full growth early in the teen years—some later—even into the early twenties. Appetite, if based on good food habits, is usually a good guide for the amounts of food needed.

The child who has furnished for him foods ample in nutritional factors, attractively yet simply served, and at regular meal intervals is indeed fortunate. Parents should provide this advantage for their child until he can maturely assume the responsibility for himself.

Using the Four Food Groups as a simple everyday guide, the individual homemaker or food service director then daily chooses her menu from the hundreds of available foods. Even so, those foods most available and best liked constitute often-repeated old favorites. Table 1 illustrates a day's choice of economical foods from the four groups, with the addition of other foods to give sufficient calories and satisfaction to the meal, as well as a reasonable amount of well-chosen fat.

The choices, with a total calorie value of 1,973, correctly approximate the caloric needs for many active women but fall below the needs of the average man. Smaller or larger servings and more or less of additional foods adjust calories to the needs of each person, for the calorie criterion is to maintain correct weight. Little children eat less; older children and teenagers eat more and larger servings. However, children and teenagers, as well as adults, should not gain excess weight.

Many foods amply provide protein both in quantity and quality, although they usually cost more than other foods. The food choices used in the example furnish both inexpensive and highly adequate protein. If a diet provides too high a calorie level, cut cost and calories by replacing some or all of the milk with reconstituted nonfat dry milk, especially for adults.

The calcium is adequate for all members of the family except in the event of rapid growth and for postmenopausal women, but additional servings of the milk group care for these conditions.

Some may consider iron the problem nutrient, since it may appear that food is inadequate in iron and hence iron medication must supplement the diet. The calculated diet furnishes 15.0 milligrams of iron—more than a man requires, which is 10.0 milligrams. This amount of iron may fall slightly below the requirement for some women, depending upon the menstrual blood loss. Actually, most drinking water and other accidental sources contain enough iron to supplement the iron in adequate food choices. It is unlikely that any normal person will become anemic if he properly chooses from the Four Food Groups. Iron pills or other medication can lead to intestinal irritation and to iron overload. Do not give iron medication to children or adults unless a physician directs, and then only for the time indicated.

Vitamin A abounds. In fact, a dark-green or deep-yellow vegetable chosen every other day and alternating with less colorful vegetables provides an abundance of this vitamin.

When one's food furnishes the three B vitamins in Table 1 (thiamine, riboflavin, and niacin) and sufficient high biologic protein (see chapters 3 and 5), all the other B vitamins are well supplied. Some foods contain preformed niacin; protein supplies the rest. The body can convert tryptophan, an essential amino acid (see chapter 3), into niacin when sufficient protein is available to the body. In the choice of foods in Table 1, the food directly supplies approximately half of the niacin, while the ample supply of high biologic protein furnishes the other half.

No problem exists regarding ascorbic acid when you include a serving of a citrus food. Many other foods form equally good sources of the vitamin, but never mistakenly assume that just any fruit, fruit drink, or fruitlike drink supplies it. (See Table 5 pages 66 and 67, for vitamin C food sources.)

Within the structure of the Four Food Groups, make any other choices from the endless variety of foods available. All regular foods fit into a group, and many less frequently used choices are equally satisfactory. If calculated, each set of choices would reveal the same two facts: (1) Food choices of the Four Food Groups can be made from all good foods; (2) These choices lead to excellent nutrition for all members of the family.

Table 1   The Nutrient Content of Foods Selected From the Four Food Groups

Food	Common Measure	Wt. in Grams	Calories kcal.	Protein gm.	Calcium mg.	Iron mg.	Vit. A IU	Thiamine mg.	Riboflavin mg.	Niacin mg.	Ascorbic Acid gm.
Fruit and Vegetable Group											
Potato, baked	1 med.	100	90	3	9	.7	trace	.10	.04	1.7	20
Cauliflower	1 cup	120	25	3	25	.8	70	.11	.10	.7	66
Orange	3-in. diam.	210	86	1	67	.3	310	.16	.06	.6	70
Apricots, dried, uncooked	¼ cup, 10 small halves	38	98	2	25	2.0	4,088	0	.06	1.2	5
Cereal and Bread Group											
Rolled oats, cooked	⅔ cup	157	87	3	14	.9	0	.13	.03	.2	0
Bread, whole-grain	2 slices	46	110	4	46	.10	trace	.12	.06	1.4	trace
Bread, 50% whole-wheat	1 slice	23	60	2	19	.6	trace	.06	.05	.6	trace
Protein Group											
Beans, common varieties, cooked	1 cup	256	230	15	74	4.6	trace	.13	.10	1.5	—
Egg	1	50	80	6	27	1.1	590	.05	.15	trace	0
Milk Group											
Milk, 2% fat	2 cups	492	290	20	704	.2	400	.20	1.04	.4	4
Totals from diet			1,156	59	1,010	12.2	5,458	1.06	1.69	8.3	165
Recommended allowance for a man (23 to 50 years old):			2,700	56	800	10	5,000	1.4	1.6	18	60
for a woman (23 to 50 years old):			2,000	44	800	18	4,000	1.0	1.2	13	60

Table 1 (cont.)   Food Additions to the Four Food Groups to Complete a Typical Day's Diet

Food	Common Measure	Wt. in Grams	Calories kcal.	Protein gm.	Calcium mg.	Iron mg.	Vit. A IU	Thiamine mg.	Riboflavin mg.	Niacin mg.	Ascorbic Acid gm.
Additions											
Margarine, oil 1st ingredient	1 tbsp.	14	100	trace	3	0	460	—	—	—	0
Oil, corn	1 tbsp.	14	125	0	0	0	—	0	0	0	0
Mayonnaise	1 tbsp.	15	110	trace	3	.1	40	trace	.01	trace	—
Lettuce	3 oz.	85	9	—	15	.4	266	.04	.04	.2	5
Tomato	1 med.	150	35	2	20	.8	1,350	.10	.06	1.0	34
Vegetable soup	1 cup	245	78	2	20	1.0	2,875	.05	.05	1.0	—
Peanut butter	1 tbsp.	16	95	4	9	.3	—	.02	.02	2.4	0
Ice cream	¼ pt.		145	3	87	—	370	.03	.13	.1	—
Wafers, sweet	2 small		120	1	9	.2	20	.01	.01	.1	0
Total from 4 food groups			1,156	59	1,010	12.2	5,458	1.06	1.69	8.3	165
Food groups diet additions			817	12	166	2.8	5,381	.25	.32	4.8	39
Totals for day's selections			1,973	71	1,176	15.0	10,839	1.31	2.01	13.1	204

* Niacin from its precursor, tryptophan.

PASTE-UP: Please put the following in place above: .....

From tryptophan of protein*   11.8
                              ――――
                               24.9

28

Chapter 2

BODY'S BIG BUSINESS

Envision the Four Food Groups as four large packages of nutrients. You interlock the four large pieces of this simple food puzzle and thus provide all units needed for building and maintaining each cell of the body. As body cells receive the materials given them by way of food, they become individual factories making and putting together puzzle pieces that we can liken to a most intricate puzzle of thousands of pieces or more. The imagination can understand only with difficulty that nutrition is both as simple as the Four Food Groups and at the same time as complex as the functions of a single body cell.

The body can properly build and maintain itself only if correct materials are available when needed. A body cell, the unit of body structure, requires at least fifty nutrients. With these nutrient units the cell makes its own structure, as well as its own hundreds of specific enzymes and coenzymes that aid the individual cell's use of nutrients. Certain cells of glands also produce necessary hormones that effectively regulate vital body functions. The body cells also make many other complex substances from the materials supplied by food, water, and air.

Metabolism

The term *metabolism* encompasses all functions of cells and their organizations (tissues and organs). *Anabolism,* the building of complex substances by cells, balances *catabolism,* the breaking down of complex substances for energy utilization and excretion of end products of metabolism. For most adults, anabolism and catabolism are equal in effect. However, in growth, pregnancy, lactation, and actual body building, the processes of anabolism are greater than those of catabolism; whereas in acute illnesses, loss of weight, and destructive conditions as a result of hormone imbalance, catabolism exceeds anabolism. In health, and with proper eating habits and exercise, metabolism amazingly holds itself in continuous balance and often does so for a lifetime.

The Nutrients and Their Functions

Most of the nutrients serve more than one function, and all are essential and available from foods of the Four Food Groups. We can list their functions under the following categories:

Nutrients That Build and Maintain Body Cells

Protein	Mineral elements
Water	Fats
Carbohydrates	

Nutrients That Regulate Body Functions

Water	Vitamins
Mineral elements	Carbohydrates, including fiber

Nutrients That Provide Energy

Carbohydrates	Fats
(starches and sugars)	Proteins

The Reconstruction of Food

Food preparation begins in the kitchen. Many foods can be served raw, others raw or cooked, while many must be cooked before certain nutrients are available and acceptable to the body. Good food preparation is both a science and an art and should capture the interest of every homemaker. First of all, learn those basic procedures assuring the best use of food without the inclusion of excess calories or loss of important nutrients. Section III discusses such basic facts and procedures for the preparation of food and its service to individuals and families. Learning to use good procedures in preparation assures that food reaches the table in its best condition for nourishing the body as well as pleasing and satisfying the diners.

Food preparation should ensure:

Food clean and safe
Proteins in their most available form.
Starches available to digestive enzymes.
Fats unharmed chemically and not soaked into starches.
Minerals retained and available.
Vitamins retained.
Cellulose softer.
Natural color retained.
Flavor retained and enhanced.
Odor pleasant and provocative to digestive response (makes the mouth water).
Food available in an attractive setting (even in a brown bag at school or on the job).

Digestion actually continues food preparation in the gastrointestinal tract. The digestive processes break down the food eaten into the nutrients suitable for entry into the bloodstream, and then and there the metabolic processes begin.

Chewing prepares food for digestion in the digestive tract, although food undergoes slight digestion in the mouth. Fortunately, you cannot swallow food easily until you chew it reasonably well, mixing it with saliva, which begins starch digestion. The stomach mixes the food with more digestive juices until it becomes quite liquid. Starches continue to digest until the contents become acid with hydrochloric acid; pepsin begins digesting protein, and rennin curds casein (a protein of milk). The fats that are already separated in particles (emulsified) may digest to some extent in the stomach also.

Most digestion occurs in the small intestine. In the presence of bile, digestive enzymes from the pancreas and the intestinal wall reduce foods to their digestive end products:

> Carbohydrates to the single sugars (glucose, fructose, and galactose).
> Fats to fatty acids and glycerol (glycerin).
> Proteins to their building block units (amino acids).

Some food material is not intended for digestion and absorption. Cellulose, or fiber, mainly stimulates the activity of the intestinal tract. The intestine normally excretes about 2 percent of the carbohydrates, 5 percent of the fats, 8 percent of the proteins of the typical mixed diet, the cellulose, and a small amount of water.

Absorption of nutrients takes place along the entire length of the small intestine. Not passively or casually, but actively, complex substances in the stomach and chemical forces in the whole digestive tract transport the nutrients across the intestinal barrier. For a number of nutrients, absorption occurs only in specified areas of the tract. Water-soluble nutrients entering the cells lining the digestive tract are transferred to blood capillaries and carried to larger and larger blood vessels, then on to the liver. Most of the fat-soluble nutrients go from digestive tract cells into the lymph, and thus indirectly into the bloodstream.

For proper nourishment, furnish the body daily with the foods of the Four Food Groups. Given the raw material, the body cares for all the intricate details involved in the acts of nutrition. Simple consideration for nutritional needs by planning around the Four Food Groups—

1. Gives sufficient nutrients (except perhaps calories or certain trace nutrients lacking in local soil or water, such as iodine and fluorine).

2. Serves as a food guide for all ages above infancy, with modification of amounts.

3. Provides the protein requirement both in quantity and quality, thus giving specific amino acids for all structures of the body, including those needed to make highly specialized substances, such as enzymes, hormones, and antibodies.

4. Furnishes adequately the less understood nutrients in biologically adequate amounts, such as vitamin B_{12}, the pyridoxines, folic acid, and certain trace minerals.

5. Automatically maintains the acid and base balance of the body.

6. Gives the correct kind and amount of fiber in the diet.

7. Adequately supplies calcium and riboflavin that can be lacking when meat constitutes the main protein food and takes the place of both the protein and milk group.

8. Makes it possible to select from the hundreds of varieties of food, thus eliminating no food nature provides.

9. Combines nutrients that facilitate assimilation and utilization of foods.

10. Gives opportunity to regulate the amount and kind of additional selected fats used.

11. Recognizes bland foods that make the diet more tolerable and provide a basis for enjoyment of colorful and flavorful foods.

12. Leaves no place for faddishness and misinformation of foods.

13. Adapts the lacto-ovo-vegetable protein diet, which provides an excellent plan for food selection.

14. Uses a simple tool in food selection of 4-4-2-2 in terms of servings or each respective group of foods.

15. Furnishes good nutrition with easily procured ordinary foods in simple programmed selection that practically assures good nutrition without threat of overnutrition or imbalance of nutrients.

16. Presents a basic dietary plan adaptable to people and their native foods throughout the world.

One can only wonder how a simple plan in food selection can assure so much in nutritional science and functional body chemistry!

From the gastrointestinal tract, the nutrients directly or indirectly issue continuously into the blood. Immediately these vital materials go to work nourishing every cell of the body. The person interested in this continuous process refers to the Four Food Groups in planning daily meals, and each day chooses a different selection of foods. Thus over a period of time he utilizes all foods, good nutrition continues, and good fellowship centers around mealtime.

AN-3

Chapter 3

THE FIRE OF LIFE

Fire, usually a terrifying word, is a welcome one in terms of body metabolism, although scientists temper the word by substituting the term *oxidation*. After using carbohydrates, fats, and proteins for building and storage, the body utilizes them for energy. This process requires a "slow burn" as the carbon materials of these nutrients combine with oxygen. The hemoglobin (a protein-iron complex) in the red blood cells carries oxygen from the lungs and releases it near every cell of the body, which accepts nutrients from the blood for fuel. The oxidation of the three nutrients releases energy, gives the body power to work, and produces heat as a by-product. The body's temperature remains at approximately 98.6 degrees Fahrenheit, and the person lives—active and capable of great potential in physical and mental work.

The Carbohydrates

Green plants use energy from the sun, water from the soil, and carbon dioxide from the air to produce sugars and starches, which provide man with the major source of his energy requirement. In the United States, carbohydrates furnish about half of the energy food of the diet. In many parts of the world, as much as four fifths of the total calories come from the starches of cereal seeds. Cereals and sugars form an acceptable, inexpensive, wholesome, and adaptable basis for other food inclusions.

Saccharide (sugar) units, composing all starches and sugars, are built by the plant in the following forms:

Sugar Units	*Examples*	*Some Food Sources*
Monosaccharides (single sugars)	Glucose (dextrose)	Many fruits and vegetables, honey, corn syrup
	Fructose (levulose)	Many fruits and vegetables, honey, corn syrup
	Galactose	Does not occur except as milk sugar (lactose) is digested
Disaccharides (two sugar units)	Sucrose	Cane, beet, and maple, sugars, fruits and vegetables

	Maltose	From malting of cereal grains
	Lactose	Milk sugar, the only carbody-drate of milk
	Starch	Cereal grains, legumes, vegetables
Polysaccharides (many sugar units)	Dextrin	Partially digested starches
	Cellulose	Fiber of fruits and vegetables, bran, coat of cereal grains
	Pectins	Animal starch, in liver and
	Glycogen	muscles

For every two units of a single sugar (monosaccharide), the plant takes out two hydrogen and one oxygen (one water molecule) molecules and bonds the two monosaccharides into one double sugar (disaccharide). As this process continues to add saccharide unit after saccharide unit, it forms large carbohydrate molecules such as starches. Thus the starchy seed or root can store potential energy for human use in a small space and in a form that offers good keeping qualities.

Eating these storehouses of energy reverses the chemical process occurring in the plant. Digestive juices furnish the water plus the specific enzymes to facilitate the process of adding water at the juncture of each two-sugar units. Hence, the saccharide units split into monosaccharides as the food reaches certain absorptive areas of the small intestine.

Do not think, however, that eating simple sugars in the first place eases metabolism. First, starches come to us by nature mixed with small but important amounts of proteins and fats, small to liberal amounts of various minerals, vitamins, and cellulose, and many of the nutrients needed for their proper use and metabolism. To eat the simple or double sugars or the pure starches exclusively would lead to the inclusion of energy food only with little of the equally important nutrients. Second, nature does not intend that we have much sugar in the diet. Not only do man and nature tend to highly refine the distinct sugars, thus giving little more than calories, but digestion of starches in foods supplies energy food to the blood rather slowly over a continuous and longer period of time. Sugars ready for absorption at once oversupply the blood as well as the metabolic facilities of the body as they work to store the sugar in the form of body starch. As a homey example, the family may like a decorative wood carrier filled with wood sitting by the fireplace, but they prefer to store the cords of wood elsewhere than in the living room. The large starch molecules tend to serve as reserve fuel that does not disturb the housekeeping (metábolism) of the body. Sugars, on the other hand, tend to be demanding at both the absorptive facilities and metabolic sites. Therefore, take most of your carbohydrates in the form of large molecules (starch). Following the Four Food Groups as a guide in meal planning automatically accomplishes this feat, providing you use additional sweet foods in moderation.

Starches and sugars are friendly nutrients and the greatest supporters of the power to do work. Since misinformation regarding these nutrients runs rampant, chapter 15 discusses common facts and fallacies regarding starches and sugars, as well as giving a correct understanding of their often mistaken role.

Since some persons should use less than the full amount of the bran portion of cereals, milled flours are commonly used. However, since the processing destroys some nutrients, the Food and Drug Administration allows enrichment of cereals and flours by the addition of thiamine, riboflavin, niacin, and iron. Enriched flour, although nutritionally preferred over unenriched flour, does not contain all the nutrients lost in milling. Enrichment does not replace whole-grain values of fiber, magnesium, zinc, folate, and vitamin B_6.

Carbohydrates make up the nutrients used in the greatest quantity by the body. Choose them mainly from whole-food sources and for the most part in the form of large molecules (the starches).

Fiber

Typical American diets notably lack fiber. A wide variety of physical complaints can be attributed to a lack of this neglected dietary item. The use of an abundance of refined cereals and breads, sugars, and fats can supply calories but no fiber. Also, few people eat liberal amounts of fruits and vegetables.

To reverse this trend, one should replace a majority of the refined foods with whole-grain cereals and breads. Vegetables and fruits also supply a liberal amount of fiber.

Cereal bran is most effective in holding water. The combination of a fiber that does not wholly disintegrate in the intestinal tract and of the water it holds gives bulk to the stool, keeps it soft, and thereby maintains normal elimination.

Although bran is the best known fiber, there are several other types of useful dietary fibers necessary for maintaining health. Pectin, lignin, and hemicellulose are examples of the fibers found in legumes, fruits, vegetables, and nuts.

When a person needs additional amounts of this digestive aid, miller's bran can be added to food. Begin with a small amount, increasing it very slowly—such as with a one teaspoon increment each day. For some, one tablespoon a day is sufficient for normal elimination. Four tablespoons is considered a maximum amount for those who require more fiber. *Bran should never be eaten dry.*

Dietary changes that increase various types of fiber often do wonders in alleviating symptoms of distress and disease. The use of laxatives and other means of forceful evacuation is debilitating and habit-forming. Fiber is a major food substance that enables the intestines to function normally.

Two dietary guides can help a person in choosing the correct foods that include fiber. One is the Four Food Groups, in which fruits, vegetables, and whole grains are listed. The other is the U.S. Dietary Goals, which advises less use of sugar and fat and greater use of the unrefined starches (whole grains and starchy vegetables). (See page 154.)

Fats

The word *fat* conveys mixed interpretations and feelings to most people—rich, good, plenty, versus unwanted, greasy, inferior. Fat is needed—is desirable—and deserves most careful consideration as a nutrient.

To make a fat molecule, three fatty acids of various-length carbon chains (four to twenty-four carbon atoms) unite with the three alcohol units of a glycerol (glycerin) molecule. At each of the three points of union one water molecule is taken out, which makes fat a high calorie nutrient. Fats can vary in nature greatly because of the many possible lengths of the carbon chain. Variation also exists in the number of places where the bonds may be doubled between carbon molecules rather than hold the greatest possible number of hydrogen atoms.

At this point, we can profitably clarify a number of terms commonly heard in discussions regarding dietary fats. All fats are made of three fatty acids and one glycerol molecule. *Saturated* fatty acids are composed of carbon chains with no double bonds between carbons and with all carbon atoms saturated with as many hydrogen atoms as the carbons can hold. In the following diagram of a portion of a saturated fatty acid, C signifies carbon, H signifies hydrogen, and O, oxygen.

Saturated fatty acids have no double bonds linking the carbons:

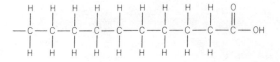

Unsaturated fatty acids have double energy bonds linking the carbons. If there is but one point of unsaturation, it is called a *monounsaturated* fatty acid, as the following portion of a fatty acid shows:

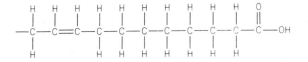

If the carbon chain contains more than one point of unsaturation, it is called a *polyunsaturated* fatty acid:

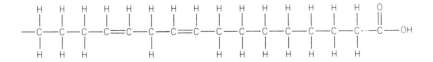

In a polyunsaturated fat, a high portion of polyunsaturated fatty acids makes up the fat. These fats tend to be oils at room temperature. One polyunsaturated fatty acid that is plentiful in seed oils—linoleic acid—is essential to good nutrition. An *essential substance* in nutrition must be obtained directly from food—the body must have this chemical structure, for the body cannot reconstruct it from similar structures.

Oils can be manufactured into a plastic or moldable solid fat for shortening, for cooking, and for margarines. During this process of *hydrogenation*, hydrogen molecules attach to some of the carbons held by double bonds, thus reducing the number of double bonds, making them single. As hydrogenation increases the saturation of a fat, it decreases the amount of linoleic acid in the oil and converts the oil into a fat that remains solid at room temperature. The following formula illustrates the process:

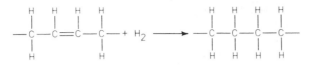

As the saturation increases and the oil becomes solid, it melts at a higher temperature than it originally did.

Dietary Goals of the United States* recommends equal amounts of saturated and polyunsaturated fatty acids in a diet in which the amount of fat does not exceed 30 percent of the total day's calories. To give the reader some idea how equal amounts of saturated and polyunsaturated fats can be accomplished in dietary planning, the following list of fatty constituents of a day's diet includes all fats used in cooking and found in prepared foods purchased:

Egg	1
Milk, 2% fat	2 cups
Margarine, liquid seed oil as the first ingredient	1 Tbsp. (level)
Oil, corn	1 Tbsp.
Peanut butter	1 Tbsp. (level)
Milk pudding or ice cream	¼ cup (level)

A diet containing only these fats has a P/S ratio of 1, which means an equal amount of saturated and polyunsaturated fat. This amount of fat is 30% of the total calories of a diet that contains approximately two thousand calories.

Fats used as fuel are almost two and one-half times more concentrated than carbohydrates and proteins. While the carbohydrates and proteins each produce four calories of heat per gram (approximately one twenty-eighth of an ounce), the fats yield nine

---

* Senate Nutrition Committee, *Dietary Goals of the United States,* revised (Washington, D.C.: 1978). Superintendent of Documents, U.S. Printing Office, 1978).

calories per gram. This means that fats yield the most energy of the three calorie-producing nutrients.

Antioxidants added to fats lengthen their keeping quality. Without this protection fats turn rancid quickly.

On the plus side of the ledger, the diet needs fats, since they are good fuel foods and carry essential fatty acids and fat-soluble vitamins. Some fat accompanying meals adds a feeling of satisfaction (satiety). Omit fats from the diet and you will experience dissatisfaction (lack of satiety).

On the negative side, fats can quickly put too many calories in the diet, leading to overweight. Since most fats and oils contain few essential nutrients, use them in moderation as a refined food. Because fats add richness to other foods, making them more appealing to most appetites, one can easily overuse them.

As a result of habit and common use, many people prefer the solid fats. In certain food preparation techniques solid fats emulsify easily through other food ingredients and are less visible, yet these solid fats are naturally low in linoleic acid or are produced by hydrogenation with a resultant loss of the polyunsaturated fatty acids.

Associated with today's affluent society is an abundance of oils manufactured into nonoily plastic, or pliable shortenings to favor the American cook's demand. Concurrent with this trend, not only does the average person eat too many fat calories, but the intake of linoleic acid is relatively low and an unfavorable picture of blood *lipids* (fats) has appeared. The greatest concern has centered around abnormally elevated blood serum *cholesterol* and *triglyceride* (fat) levels. Cholesterol, normally present and needed in all tissues of the body, is a type of solid alcohol related to fat. Blood serum triglyceride levels measure the actual pure fats in the blood. An abnormally high concentration of these substances has been associated with coronary heart attacks called *infarct* and other related conditions of circulatory deterioration.

Fats that enter the body's circulation are not water soluble. In order to be transported, these fats must be combined with protein, which is soluble. There are different "packs" of *lipoproteins* (fat-proteins). Some are fats of high density (HDL), and some of low density (LDL). The high density packs are associated with a low risk of heart attacks. Researchers are studying the HDL fraction to determine whether or not these fats are truly protective, and if so, how they can be best increased. Physical activity appears to be an important way to increase the HDL.

While science offers no direct proof that a person will avoid early heart attacks by merely altering the amount and kind of fat in the diet, the indirect proof is overwhelming. *Atherosclerosis,* a slowly developing disease of the arteries, begins with a thickening of the inner lining of the blood vessels from one to many layers of cells. Then various materials, including cholesterol, are deposited, and the blood vessel area narrows; meanwhile the vessel walls lose their elasticity. Even three of the following high risk factors present in an individual indicate needed dietary control. Better still, dietary control early in life before certain of these factors develop may be of utmost value.

The high risk factors:
> Being a man (more subject to heart attacks than are premenopausal women).
> Hereditary factors (following family trends, owing to genetic differences).
> Little exercise.
> Inner stress.
> Elevated blood cholesterol level.
> High blood pressure.
> Overweight.
> Cigarette smoking.
> Excessive coffee drinking.
> Insufficient sleep.

Dietary control includes lowering total dietary fat in the typical American diet. This diet often contains 45 to 55 percent or more of its calories in fat. A diet in which fat composes no more than 30 percent of the calories shows promise of better balance. You should carefully select separated fats (oils) so that they include ample amounts of linoleic acid unchanged by hydrogenation. Maintain an equal relationship of polyunsaturated fats to saturated fats in the diet. Reserve the saturated fats to a limited amount of dairy and egg fats, for they carry other essential nutrients, such as fat-soluble vitamins. Add small amounts of seed oils and you will then provide this one-to-one relationship, yet can keep the total amount of fat low.

Figure 1 shows percentages of linoleic acid in a number of fats and oils of plant and animal origin. Careful study shows that animal fats as a whole contain less of this essential fatty acid than do some of the vegetable fats. Safflower, corn, soy, and cottonseed oils provide readily available supplies of linoleic acid. Soft margarines on the market today containing liquid seed oils have higher percentages of linoleic acid than the solid stick margarines indicated in Figure 1.

Strictly avoid the temptation to overuse even the desirable oils, but for the most part, choose the little separated fat you do use from the oils that supply linoleic acid.

Figure 1

Percent of linoleic acid in fats and oils of plant and animal origin. (From Coons, in the *Journal of the American Dietetic Association,* 34:[1958]:242. Courtesy of the American Dietetic Association.)

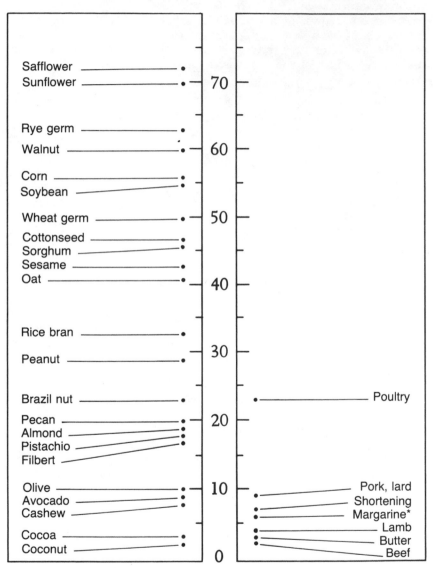

* Margarines containing liquid seed oils are higher in linoleic acid.

Also include in the diet some of the saturated short-chained fatty acids that carry fat-soluble nutrients. A limited number of eggs, some milk fat, or fortified margarine with liquid oil as the first or second stated ingredient enhances the diet and gives a balance of fatty acids. Although egg yolks contain high amounts of cholesterol, they carry substances that aid the body in properly utilizing fats. Furthermore, some evidence indicates that the body does not absorb all dietary cholesterol. Some studies show that the body absorbs only one and one-half times the square root of the ingested (eaten) cholesterol. (See article by Ancel Keys, "Blood Lipids in Man—A Brief Review," in *Journal of the American Dietetic Association,* December, 1967.) Hence, it appears that a moderate cholesterol intake for the normal person is not undesirable, but that a higher intake is not recommended.

A lacto-ovo-vegetable diet may contain, in one day, two cups of 1 percent fat milk, a serving of creamed cottage cheese (or a small serving of American cheese), one egg, or one-fourth pint of ice cream. This choice of food gives less than 300 milligrams of cholesterol from food sources for the day—a low amount of dietary cholesterol. The United States Dietary Goals suggests that cholesterol consumption be limited to 300 milligrams a day. According to the theory of cholesterol absorption stated in the preceding paragraph, most people will absorb less than twenty-six milligrams of cholesterol from these dietary inclusions. Many diets that daily contain eggs and meats—especially organ meats—regularly include as much as one thousand milligrams of cholesterol each day. But most people can handle efficiently the cholesterol of three or four eggs a week and will benefit from the nutrients provided.

Certain general recommendations have emerged from the study of types of fats and fatty acids in nutrition: (1) a diet containing 40 percent fat calories or more is undoubtedly too high in fat and should be lowered; (2) the daily diet should include some unhydrogenated (unhardened) seed oils; and (3) though highly saturated in nature, short-carbon-chained fats in egg yolk and milk fat are of value in human nutrition when used moderately.

The ratio of polyunsaturated fat to saturated fat in the diet has arrested the interest of nutritionists and thoughtful laypersons. Both types of fatty acids are needed, but nutritionists generally agree that certain relationships between the two are more desirable than others.

Diets in which the fatty foods include only dairy and egg fats, meat fats from hard animal fats, and hydrogenated oils contain few polyunsaturates. The average American diet tends to have a very low

P/S ratio. This is illustrated in the following fat-containing foods of a day's diet:

Milk, whole	3 cups
Egg	1
Butter	2 Tbsp.
Cream, whipping	2 Tbsp.
Beef hamburger, regular	3 oz.
Shortening	2 Tbsp.

P/S ratio 0.04 (1.0 to 0.04—only 0.04 gram polyunsaturated fat to each gram of saturated fat).

By changing two items in the menu, the P/S ratio can be somewhat improved:

Butter to margarine in which the first stated ingredient is liquid seed oil

Beef hamburger, regular, to beef hamburger, lean

P/S ratio 0.61 (1.0 to 0.61)

Dairy fats that contain important fat-soluble vitamins can be included in the diet and one still attain a good P/S ratio if a vegetable protein food replaces red meat:

Milk, whole	3 cups
Egg	1
Margarine, liquid seed oil first stated ingredient	2 Tbsp.
Cream, whipping	2 Tbsp.
Beef- or chicken- style soy product	3 oz.
Oil, corn	2 Tbsp.

P/S ratio 1.33 (1.0 to 1.33)

For the person whose physician advises a diet very low in saturated fatty acids, the latter list can be adjusted to low-fat milk, only egg white, and no whipping cream or if allowed a small amount of evaporated milk in its place.

Such a diet has fewer calories. If the person needs more calories they should be supplied by increasing the amount of large-molecule carbohydrates (potatoes, whole-grain cereals, et cetera) eaten.

The day's menu on page 24 gives a P/S ratio of 1. This means that for every gram of saturated fat eaten, there is a gram of polyunsaturated fat. This ratio is highly recommended for the average healthy American.

Careful food selection accomplishes three points worthy of consideration:

1. It decreases the total fat of the typical American diet.

2. It increases the relationship of linoleic acid to saturated fatty acids.

3. The diet contains familiar foods without omitting any food group.

For now, the weight of evidence of dietary change for the average American and other peoples for whom coronary heart disease poses a serious threat shows the beneficial effects of dietary shift in favor of a slightly higher amount of polyunsaturates in fatty acids, but this does not mean that one should eliminate all the saturated fats from the diet. It may be that this dietary shift should be made very early in life, for it could mean maximum benefit in a longer life, with the vascular system showing less damage with increasing years.

By definition, three fatty acids plus one glycerol compose all fats. The stomach and, more specifically, the small intestine digest these fats into smaller components by means of specific enzymes. Some foods have small amounts of monoglycerides and diglycerides added; the label declares such. These additions give a soft spreadability to certain fats and also furnish a greater range in temperature tolerance from a warm room to refrigeration. They are merely partially digested fats that are acceptable to the digestive tract along with other fats. As these digested products pass through the intestinal wall they form again into simple fats, which the lymph picks up and carries to the blood. Although fat serves primarily as an energy food, it also provides support, insulation, and contouring of the "well-engineered" curves of the body.

Proteins and the Amino Acids

Proteins received their names from Greek and mean "to take first place." As nutrients, they not only furnish energy but actively build living nitrogenous tissue. The nitrogen of proteins makes them differ from the carbohydrates and fats, and because proteins, first of all, build body protoplasm, their position as first is seldom challenged.

Amino acids make up proteins and constitute the very building blocks of the living cell. Twenty-two amino acids occur both in foods and in body proteins, and although no food protein exactly resembles body proteins, food does furnish all the amino acids from which the body selects those needed to make each of its own many specific protein substances. Like the units of carbohydrates and fats, protein units are put together in food—the units being amino acids. Removal of water between each two units forms a large protein molecule containing hundreds of amino acids. During digestion, highly specialized enzymes in the stomach and intestine split the protein molecule with water at the junctions of amino acids until they are the size and nature the blood can absorb.

Given enough nitrogen-containing foods as well as sufficient total food, the body constructs some of the amino acids lacking from the food but required by the tissues. Adults, however, require nine *essential* amino acids. This term indicates that the body must obtain them structurally complete directly from food. These amino acids are: isoleucine, leucine, lysine, methionine, phenylalanine, threonine, tryptophan, valine, and histidine. Infants and children also need arginine.

A food containing amino acids in proportions and amounts needed by the body is considered a *complete* protein, or a protein of *high biologic value*. Examples of such proteins are milk, milk products, eggs, meat, fish, and poultry.

When a food lacks or has too little of one or more of the essential amino acids, it cannot of itself meet the needs of the tissues. Because such foods can only partially fill the protein needs, they are called *incomplete* proteins, or proteins of *low biologic value*. The legumes have notably low amounts of methionine, and the cereals little lysine. Besides being low in lysine, rice has little threonine; cornmeal and corn cereals are low in both tryptophan and lysine.

Complete protein foods, however, can effectively supplement the incomplete. Also a surprisingly good amount of supplementation results by serving two unlike, incomplete proteins together. Some admirable food habits have aided the human race in survival: the combination of milk with cereal, the eating of corn and beans together, and the use of rice with beans. Soybeans, because of their high protein content, are important legumes, and their products function very closely to a protein of high biologic value. One important consideration in supplementation is that foods furnishing different missing amino acids must be absorbed into the bloodstream at nearly the same time, for the cells that do the tissue building must have all their materials at the time they are needed. If the building is detained for long because of lacking materials, the whole project is scrapped, thus tending toward stunted growth and other signs of malnutrition. Many peoples have good and vital food habits. Never disturb cultural mores in food unless better ones are both available and acceptable to the peoples involved.

Table 2   Protein From Some Common Food Sources

Food	Amount	Protein gm.
Milk, fluid, whole	1 cup (8 oz.)	9
2% fat	1 cup	9
nonfat	1 cup	9
evaporated, unsweetened, undiluted	½ cup	9
dry, nonfat, instant	¼ cup	8
Buttermilk, cultured	1 cup	9
Cheese, cheddar or American	1-in. cube	4
Cheese foods, cheddar	1 oz.	6
Cottage cheese, creamed	¼ cup	8
uncreamed	¼ cup	10
Cream cheese	1 oz.	2
Ice cream, plain	½ cup	3
Ice milk	½ cup	4
Yogurt	1 cup	8
Egg	1	6
Beans, mature (common varieties), cooked	1 cup	15
Peas, split, dry, cooked	½ cup	10
Peanut butter	1 tbsp.	4
Almonds, shelled	1 oz.	5
Cashew nuts	1 oz.	5
Coconut, fresh, shredded	¼ cup	1
Peanuts	1 oz.	8
Pecan halves	¼ cup	3
Walnuts, English, halves	¼ cup	4
Breads, various kinds, griddle cakes	1 slice or serving	2
Cereals, ready-to-eat	1-oz. serving	1-3
Cereals, cooked	1 cup	3-5
Wheat germ	1 tbsp.	1
Fruits and vegetables, most varieties	1 serving	1-3
Gluten, wheat, prepared	1 serving	approx. 7
Nutmeat analog, dark, solid	½-in. slice	approx. 15
Nutmeat analog, light, solid	½-in. slice	approx. 9
Soy vegetable protein: chicken, beef, and ham styles	3 oz.	18
Meat equivalents for comparison: Chicken, boneless	3 oz.	18
beef, steak	3 oz.	20-24
ham	3 oz.	18

Pages 152, 153 give the recommended daily allowances of protein for age, sex, and condition as listed by the Food and Nutrition Board of the National Research Council. Food composition tables, such as *Nutritive Value of American Foods,* U.S. Department of Agriculture Handbook No. 456, help calculate the intake of protein as well as other nutrients, and serve as valuable references. However, for proper everyday use, the Four Food Groups lead all members of the family to the inclusion of foods that fill the need for protein both in quantity and quality. Food group selections as calculated on pages 27, 28 provide 59 grams of protein. This amount of protein is easily obtained by giving proper thought to the Four Food Groups in meal planning. Eating more or less total food makes it possible for each member of the family to have the amount of protein he needs. When food additions are added (p. 28) to include sufficient calories, the total amount of protein is 71 grams, which is adequate for a pregnant woman.

Table 2 gives the common food sources of protein for convenient reference.

Digestion of proteins begins in the stomach and ends in the intestinal tract. Protein-splitting enzymes are highly specific in their work of preparing the amino acid building blocks for passage through the intestinal barrier and into the bloodstream. From this rapidly moving transport system, the cells pick up what they need to produce any enzymes, hormones, antibodies, or other protein structures that have a specific, vital function. The work of the cells is simple if the materials are on hand, but substitutions are difficult to make, often unsatisfactory, and possibly entirely unusable.

After the cells select what amino acids they need, the unused ones, as well as those replaced by new material, return to the liver, which sheers off the nitrogen portion of the amino acids and changes it to urea. The blood takes this end product of metabolism to the kidneys, which promptly eliminate the excess urea in the urine. Urea is the largest solid excretory product dissolved in the urine, although small amounts of other nitrogen products are also excreted. For instance, the body excretes creatinine in proportion to the amount of active nitrogen tissue living in the body from day to day.

The recommended daily allowances state the amount of protein needed each day; the Four Food Groups plan translates this requirement into terms of everyday food. Thus the body functions efficiently, for it has what it requires when needed without the possibility of under- or over-protein nutrition.

Energy Metabolism

Proteins are primarily used to build, whereas carbohydrates and fats are used primarily for energy. Eventually, proteins are burned for energy to the extent of four calories per gram as are the carbohydrates. Fats yield nine calories per gram. The body is in energy balance when the calories eaten equal the calories expended in work or growth. Too few calories lead to weight loss; too many, to weight gain.

AN-4

Chapter 4

IN THE ASHES

Foods that supply energy are not composed purely of carbohydrate, fat, and protein. Nature combines the energy foods with many other nutrients. When the body oxidizes calorie foods for energy, it leaves ash materials, or those nutrients that remain essentially unchanged. These minerals exist in food as various forms of mineral salts. The most common mineral salt is sodium chloride, or table salt. Even though many minerals are needed for the nutritional processes of the body, they are retained in small amounts. Only 4 percent of the body's weight consists of mineral salts, found in both the hard and soft tissues of the body as well as its fluids.

After burning foods in the laboratory, scientists can analyze the ash to determine the mineral composition of each food. Food composition tables give the amounts of various minerals found in foods. These minerals are packaged together in foods in such a way that it is usually necessary to account for but two—calcium and iron. You can achieve this security quite automatically by planning the diet according to the Four Food Groups, making it unnecessary to check on each nutrient.

In certain geographical areas the diet may lack some trace minerals, and two minerals, iodine and fluorine, should be provided in ways approved by public health authorities in those areas where the water or soil does not furnish them in the minute quantities needed by the body.

All foods of the Four Food Groups contribute toward the mineral requirements of the body. Some are major sources, some minor. Some foods that contribute a major amount of certain minerals may have little of others. Milk, a major source of calcium and phosphorus, contributes very little toward the iron requirement of the body. No single food eaten regularly provides a large portion of the iron requirement. Rather, a number of foods contribute small but worthwhile amounts of iron to make up the day's requirement. Cereals, fruits, and vegetables all add to the iron pool, but seldom could their contribution of calcium give sufficient of this mineral to assure good nutrition.

Calcium

Except when growth, pregnancy, or lactation and postmenopause makes extra demands, two cups of milk daily will meet the calcium requirement. Other food groups contribute small amounts of calcium but seldom enough to complete the daily requirement.

Milk is an excellent source of calcium, and all forms of milk provide equally efficient amounts in a well-utilized form—fresh whole, low-fat, skim, dry, evaporated, buttermilk, yogurt, or any of the acid milks. Commercially fortified soy beverage is another excellent source of calcium. Ice cream contributes calcium but is not a major source because desserts should be used infrequently and in relatively small portions.

A large serving (at least one full cup) of such greens as collards, kale, turnip, and mustard provides about as much calcium as one cup of milk. Cabbage, broccoli, and cauliflower contribute lesser amounts of calcium but more than most other vegetables. Some vegetables have calcium in the oxalate salt form, thus rendering the mineral quite unavailable so that little or none is absorbed. Spinach, beet greens, chard, and New Zealand spinach do not have much available calcium. However, do not avoid these greens, for they contain other valuable nutrients. Milk can efficiently provide calcium along with other nutrients important in bone building and upkeep.

An occasional fruit or vegetable may be a good source of calcium, but the menu maker must ask the question fairly, "How much do I serve of this food and how often?" Provide vital nutrients from foods regularly eaten rather than rationalize an alternate that you might use only on occasion. A serving once a week of a green vegetable containing the equivalent calcium of one cup of milk would replace but one cup of milk once a week. The fact that an occasionally served food is a good source of calcium does not give license to omit milk from the diet. Young children, who need calcium in amounts equal to adults, cannot eat the bulk of vegetable foods required to meet their need for this mineral. Teenagers, who need more calcium than adults, scarcely can or will eat sufficient amounts of vegetable food daily.

Calcium, needed by the bones for their structure, is also vital for the moment-by-moment maintenance of life. Such vital functions as heartbeat and normal clotting of blood depend upon the correct amount of calcium in the blood. Since the bones act as an emergency source of calcium for vital uses, a dietary deficiency may go unrecognized for many years. Serious decalcification of bones may be the first symptom, discovered only after a weakened bone fracture.

Recent studies show that postmenopausal women who have followed the lacto-ovo-vegetarian diet for at least twenty years do not lose bone mineral to the extent that closely paired nonvegetarian women do. The vegetarians lost 18 percent of their bone mineral upon aging, while the nonvegetarian women lost 35 percent. On the average, elderly nonvegetarian women were in the "fracture region" of bone mineral loss, whereas the vegetarian women's bones would not fracture easily.

Many authorities in bone demineralization now recommend that premenopausal women should have 1000 milligrams of calcium a day and postmenopausal women 1200 to 1500 milligrams.

Table 3 reveals the importance of milk and milk products as a source of calcium; it also shows other foods that contribute to the calcium needs of the body.

Iron

The study of iron as a nutrient presents many facets of interest. The entire body contains only one tenth of an ounce. Iron is present in every cell of the body, although the hemoglobin in the blood ties up approximately two thirds of it. Oxidation, or use of the carbohydrates, fats, and proteins, could not take place without an iron complex carrying oxygen to the cells, and iron within the cells receiving the vital oxygen.

Iron, unlike calcium and many other minerals, is not excreted readily when excessive amounts build up in the blood. To safeguard against the possibility of iron toxicity, specialized proteins in the intestinal tract under normal conditions regulate the intake of iron into the blood. The amount of iron absorption can be more or less, depending upon the body's need at the time. On the average, the body absorbs only one tenth of the iron intake. As little as this is (about one to one and a half milligrams), it equals what is lost in urine and sweat.

The woman's monthly cycle adds greatly to the iron requirement, and although menstrual iron loss varies greatly, on the average a daily intake of five to ten milligrams of iron in addition to the regular nutritional requirement for the mineral will replace the loss. Because pregnancy and lactation carry approximately an equal requirement for iron, the woman needs extra iron from the onset of menstruation until the menopause.

Egg yolk, legumes, whole grains, enriched flours, breads, and cereals regularly contribute iron. Dark-green leafy vegetables, dried fruits, and dark molasses constitute especially good sources, but in many diets are used so infrequently that they contribute only minor amounts. When cast-iron cooking utensils were used regularly, iron deficiency was rare.

Only when most of the calories of the day come from the foods of the Four Food Groups are the iron requirements met. In many diets a large portion of the calories comes from various sugars, refined starches, and separated fats as found in sweet rolls, potato chips, and candies. Such diets can scarcely contain enough iron to replace body losses and meet growth requirements. Especially is this true for women, children, and teenage girls. Women who have a heavy menstrual flow and who have reproductive nutritional stress may require iron supplements in small amounts—even under "normal" conditions.

Table 4 shows the iron distribution in many natural foods. By including a wide selection of foods, you can meet the iron requirement.

Iodine

Most areas have sufficient iodine in the soil, but "goiter regions" do occur in many parts of the world, leading to the common occurrence of serious deficiency symptoms. In these areas, public health measures must supply this vital mineral. When the body lacks the necessary trace amounts of iodine, it cannot maintain proper regulation of metabolism. This condition may lead to serious developmental retardation in prenatal life or to mental and physical decline in childhood and adult years.

The use of iodized salt in cooking and at the table most satisfactorily supplies this mineral. When a physician advises a low sodium (salt) diet for indefinite periods of time, he should provide his patient with another source of the mineral if he lives in one of the goiter regions of the world, unless he has access to sufficient food imported from nongoiter regions.

Fluorine

Some underground waters as they pass over fluorine-containing rocks dissolve traces of the mineral. When the proportion reaches 1.0 to 1.2 parts of fluorine to 1 million parts water, the mineral greatly aids in strong tooth and bone formation and maintenance. Such teeth are highly resistant to caries.

Since much of the drinking water contains no fluorine, large communities in flouride-deficient areas now fluoridate the water supply. This inexpensive and safe method of lessening tooth decay is especially effective in prenatal development and the early years of childhood. If no fluorine is available naturally or artificially in the water supply, the physician or dentist can supply this trace mineral by other means. Adults also profit nutritionally from the correct amount of fluorides, especially as it may lessen weakening of the bones in old age. Multiple sources of fluorides should not be used. For instance, if the water contains fluoride naturally or is fluoridated, do not give children a fluoride supplement.

Other Microminerals

Other microminerals are also essential to the metabolism of carbohydrates, proteins, and fats. Zinc and chromium are necessary for the passage of glucose from the blood into many body cells. Zinc is a component of at least twenty enzymes that contain metals, and these enzymes function in many vital ways. Chromium enhances the activity of several enzymes, including the hormone insulin. These microminerals are examples of a number of other minerals that serve in vital functions in micro amounts. They are supplied by food when a variety of foods is chosen from all the food groups. Most of these micronutrients are provided abundantly when liberal amounts of whole grains, legumes, and nuts are included in the diet.

Water

Because every nutrient is vital, it is without point to compare the nutrients in this respect. Water, however, carries all nutrients and end products of metabolism. Water composes two thirds of the body weight. In positive health, water is in balance inside and outside every living cell.

Many people starve the body of water. Too little water intake can cause intestinal stagnation and can require a compensation of practically every cell of the body to "make do" on less water than it needs. Sugar-laden (or artificially sweetened) and caffeine-spiked drinks do not take the place of plain water. The sugar, chemicals, and drugs merely add to the problems of the body's adjustment to less of what it needs and more of what it has to contend with. The answer to "I'm thirsty, what can I have to drink?" is *water*. A water-deprived body is often a tired body.

The body obtains water from food containing liquid, from drinks, and from oxidation of all foods. When the body burns food, it produces each day more than one cup of water. Take plenty of good water as water, liberally, and especially between meals. Adults should put water drinking into their dietary habits, and should also make water

Table 3   Calcium From Some Common Food Sources

Food	Amount	Calcium mg.
Milk		
Fluid, whole	1 cup	288
nonfat	1 cup	298
Buttermilk, from skim milk	1 cup	298
Evaporated, undiluted	1 cup	635
Dry, nonfat, instant	1 cup	905
Cheese		
Cheddar or American	1-in. cube	128
Cheese foods, cheddar	1 oz.	162
Cottage cheese, creamed	½ cup	106
uncreamed	½ cup	101
Milk Beverages and Desserts		
Cocoa	1 cup	286
Malted milk	1 cup	364
Cornstarch pudding	1 cup	290
Custard, baked	1 cup	278
Ice cream, plain	¼ pt. (or ½ cup)	87
Ice milk	½ cup	146
Yogurt	1 cup	295
Mature Beans (Legumes), Nuts		
Almonds	¼ cup	83
Beans, dry (common varieties), cooked	1 cup	74
Brazil nuts	¼ cup	65
Vegetables		
Broccoli spears, cooked	1 cup	132
Cabbage, cooked	1 cup	75
Cabbage, pakchoi (nonheading green-leaf type), cooked	1 cup	222
Collards, cooked	1 cup	289
Dandelion greens, cooked	1 cup	252
Kale, cooked	1 cup	147
Mustard greens, cooked	1 cup	193
Spinach, cooked	1 cup	167
Turnip greens, cooked	1 cup	267
Fruits		
Dates, dry, pitted, cut	½ cup	52
Figs, 1½-inch diameter	3	40
Raisins, dried	½ cup	50

Table 4   Iron From Some Common Food Sources

Food	Amount	Iron mg.
Milk	1	1.1
Meat, lean	3 oz.	approx. 3.0
Mature Beans and Peas (Legumes), Nuts		
Almonds, Brazil nuts, cashew nuts, walnuts	¼ cup	approx. 1.5
Beans (common varieties), cooked, drained	1 cup	4.9
Lentils, cooked	1 cup	3.2
Peas, dry, cooked	1 cup	4.2
Vegetables		
Lima Beans, immature, cooked	1 cup	4.3
Carrots, cauliflower, sweet corn	1 cup	approx. 1.0
Greens, cooked	1 cup	approx. 2.5-4.0
Peas, green, cooked	1 cup	2.9
Sweet potato	1 med. lg.	1.0
Tomato, cooked	1 cup	1.2
Fruits		
Apricots and peaches, dried, cooked	1 cup	5.1
Berries, fresh	1 cup	approx. 1.5
Dates, dry, cut	½ cup	2.6
Grape juice	1 cup	0.8
Prunes, dried, softened	4 medium	1.1
Prune juice, canned	1 cup	10.5
Raisins, dried	½ cup	2.8
Watermelon	wedge 4″ × 8″	2.1
Grain Products		
Bread, enriched	1 slice	approx. 0.6
Flour and meal, whole or enriched, dry	¼ cup	approx. 1.0
Spaghetti and macaroni, enriched, dry	⅓ cup	approx. 1.0
Wheat germ	¼ cup	1.8
Syrup, dark	1 tbsp.	approx. 1.0
Sugar, brown	1 tbsp.	.5

readily available to little children so that they can form good water-drinking habits early in life.

Most minerals are readily available from the foods of the Four Food Groups. You can readily supply those that may require special consideration, such as iodine and fluorine, by following the instructions of local public health authorities. Neither old nor young should overlook the water requirements of the body.

Chapter 5

EVERYBODY LOVES A VITAMIN

At the turn of this century the word *vitamin* did not exist. When Dr. Casimir Funk discovered that food contained minute substances that were not minerals or calorie nutrients but were vital to life, he considered them vital amines (proteins). In 1911 he named these substances "vitamines." Soon after this date it was demonstrated that different vitamines specifically prevented and cured certain diseases that had plagued the peoples of the world for centuries.

In the 1930s and 1940s these vital nutrients were rediscovered from the standpoint of their chemical composition and function. The name had lost its final *e* and was now *vitamin*. By the time the vitamins no longer mystified, the wonder was "How can all vitamins be classed under one name?" Chemically they differ greatly and run the gamut of many types of organic compounds. Few relate to proteins in any way.

The changing of the name by dropping the one vowel sufficed, for it indicated that vitamins were just *vitamins* and no longer closely associated with the proteins, and the public neither wanted nor needed any other classification. Everyone loved the vitamins. Everyone hoped that scientists would discover other vitamins that would prevent other dreaded diseases. The vitamin pill charlatans moved in almost as fast as vitamins were synthesized commercially. The vitamin-conscious decades followed.

Today the study of vitamins still challenges, but now the concern is how the body uses these vitamins and how they relate to the use of the other nutrients. It is now known that all vitamins, in the quite small amounts required to saturate body tissues, function as coenzymes or hormonelike compounds. Additional amounts may be neither beneficial nor desirable. Excessive amounts of some vitamins are toxic. If you choose intelligently from the Four Food Groups, you will eat a balance of nutrients.

The earliest classification of vitamins still remains their chief organization: the fat-soluble and the water-soluble. This classification roughly tells where a vitamin can be found, how well it resists oxidation or destructive change, and to some extent, whether or not the body stores it.

There are four recognized fat-soluble vitamins: A, D, E, and K. Eleven substances known as the B-complex vitamins and vitamin C constitute the water-soluble vitamins. Five B-complex vitamins form parts of coenzymes and render vital services to the metabolic processes essential to the utilization of carbohydrates, fats, and proteins. These vitamins are thiamine (B_1), riboflavin (B_2), niacin, the pyridoxines (B_6), and pantothenic acid. Two of the B vitamins, B_{12} and folic acid, are essential to the blood-making organs of the body. Also, vitamin B_{12} is essential to normal nerve response. Four vitaminlike compounds require no special dietary concern as they are readily made from other available compounds, or synthesized by bacteria in the intestinal tract, or not proved essential in human nutrition. These four vitamins are choline, biotin, para-aminobenzoic acid, and inositol.

Vitamin C, known as ascorbic acid, is essential for a number of vital metabolic processes. This vitamin keeps the tissues of the body intact and, in ways different from the B vitamins, facilitates the oxidation and reduction processes of energy metabolism.

As with all the other nutrients, a well-chosen daily diet from the Four Food Groups liberally supplies the needed vitamins. Substituting foods from one group for another will not assure the diet of all the nutrients. Heeding the special instructions of the fruit and vegetable group (to include a green or yellow vegetable and a citrus fruit) assures vitamins A and C, because it is possible to choose fruits and vegetables with minimal amounts and bypass the better sources of both vitamins.

A brief review of the vitamins shows how specific food sources are included in order to compose a diet adequate for all the body's functions.

The Fat-soluble Vitamins

Each of the fat-soluble vitamins exists in several nutritionally active forms, each with its own name and specific chemical structure. No one name would describe all its forms any more than would the name of a twin or a triplet refer to each individual in the group. Because of this, chemical names are not commonly used, but rather a "tag name" of an initial indicating the whole related group.

Vitamin A
Foods of vegetable origin do not contain vitamin A. Rather,

certain yellow pigments of the carotenes in green and yellow foods serve as precursors of vitamin A. The intestinal wall can convert four carotenes into vitamin A.

Preformed vitamin A occurs only in foods of animal origin, because animals convert carotenes capable of forming vitamin A and dissolve them in certain fat-containing tissues and animal products. Thus butterfat, egg yolk, and their products supply this vitamin, as well as certain animal tissues such as liver.

Although the body utilizes preformed vitamin A more efficiently than the carotenes, a well-constructed diet derives most of its vitamin A from carotene sources. New knowledge gives added reason to include an abundance of the carotenes as one of the "protective nutrients." The animal sources if used alone would produce a diet too high in fat, cholesterol, and other fat-related substances for wise food choices. Therefore, it is important to rely partially on the dark-green and deep-yellow vegetables. One serving daily of a green or yellow vegetable with the other food inclusions of the Four Food Groups amply supplies this vitamin.

Understanding the natural abundance of carotene-containing foods makes it difficult to believe that many diets lack vitamin A. But because so many people have not learned to like a wide variety of vegetables, they often shortchange vitamin A in their diet. Include a variety of vegetables in the diets of young children—giving them tiny amounts (even fractions of a teaspoonful) with well-liked foods when they are hungry and continuing often until they acquire an acceptance. It pleases any hostess to have everyone at the table enthusiastically receive the vegetables served.

Carotene is not easily destroyed, but choose fresh vegetables in prime condition. Carotene can be lost through oxidation (exposure to air or overcooking), but properly prepared food retains it.

A severe loss of vitamin A (as well as all fat-soluble vitamins) occurs through the use of mineral oil as a laxative. Therefore, never use such a nutritionally dangerous product as a home remedy. Mineral oil is not a food oil; it is not digested; it is not absorbed by the intestine. It does have some of the characteristics of a food oil; one is its ability to absorb fat-soluble substances, which it does not release, but are lost in the intestinal excretions. A child, especially, when given mineral oil regularly can become severely deficient in fat-soluble vitamins.

Deficiency symptoms of the vitamins are legion, and this book cannot possibly describe in detail the effects of vitamin deficiency on the body. In general, vitamin A deficiency adversely affects many functions of the body and appears especially in poor hair and skin conditions and growth abnormalities. A deficiency of vitamin A also affects the health of all living tissues of body orifices by the loss of tissue ability to remain normally moist or lubricated. Also the eye may lose its ability to adapt quickly from light to dark (night blindness). Serious and continued deficiency causes blindness, owing to the disease xerophthalmia (meaning "dry eyes").

The Four Food Groups used as a basis for meal planning assure plenty of vitamin A. It can be obtained preformed in milk, milk products, and eggs or in previtamin form from the green and yellow vegetables. Green vegetables also contain the yellow pigment, but the darker green pigment, chlorophyll, masks it.

It is easy for individuals or whole families to slip into the habit of bypassing the very-green and very-yellow vegetables, and especially is this so with teenage boys. At the very time the health of the skin is paramount, unfortunately teen young people lose interest in the foods that best supply the vitamins needed by the skin for its complicated functions.

In the 1980 revision of the recommended dietary allowances, vitamin A is given in retinal equivalents rather than in international units. The amount needed per day does not differ from the former recommendations of five thousand IU for men and four thousand IU for women.

Vitamin E

A normal good diet including a liberal amount of whole grains supplies sufficient vitamin E, called the tocopherols. Wheat-germ oil provides a concentrated form of this vitamin.

Large amounts of polyunsaturated fats increase the requirement of this vitamin, and although the body requires linoleic acid (the essential polyunsaturated fatty acid), do not use it excessively. This fact points up the overruling principle of moderation in all matters relating to nutrition.

Vitamin K

The "koagulation vitamin," discovered by Henrik Dam, of Copenhagen, in 1935, is essential to normal blood clotting. Present in very small amounts in leafy vegetables, egg yolk, soybean oil, and liver, under correct conditions it is also synthesized in the intestinal tract.

Physicians prescribe vitamin K for some newborns and for certain abnormal conditions. In fact, the knowledge of this vitamin and its use in medical practice is extremely important in saving lives of individuals with certain types of hemorrhage.

Under normal conditions, the body has sufficient vitamin K. Under certain abnormal conditions, one may need additional vitamin K, but only with medical supervision, for overdosage is toxic.

Vitamin D

Sufficient vitamin D prevents the bone disease rickets. This vitamin aids in the proper absorption and utilization of calcium and phosphorus in bone building and exists in two principal forms. One is preformed in certain animal fats (some fish livers, notably), and the other is the result of irradiation of ultraviolet light (certain wavelengths of sunlight) on some plant materials. Both are effective.

The human being can make a vitamin D by exposure of the skin to sunlight. Since it is difficult to regulate the amount synthesized from a type of cholesterol in the skin, the amount from this source may or may not suffice—depending on climatic conditions, personal habits of living, and the amount of skin pigmentation.

It is most practical to give babies, young children, and pregnant and lactating mothers a vitamin D source as prescribed by a physician. If necessary he can also prescribe for older children. Adults have no specific requirement for this vitamin, but dairy and egg fats assure a small intake.

Severe toxicity may result from overdoses of vitamin D. Always follow instructions exactly in giving vitamin D, and use only the vitamin D supplements prescribed by the physician. He should know, for instance, whether or not you use vitamin D fortified milk and whether or not the child has regular exposure to the sun. Strictly avoid sunburning, for it damages the skin and provides no nutritional advantage.

Ten micrograms of vitamin D is four hundred international units.

The Water-soluble Vitamins

Vitamin C and the various B vitamins are water-soluble. As a rule vitamins in this group are easily lost in one or more ways. First of all, because a water media carries them, they can be lost when cooking water is not utilized. Larger food pieces and a short cooking time lessen inevitable loss of these vulnerable vitamins. Good cooks use enough water for rapid heat transfer but not enough to necessitate draining after cooking. Cooking with unneutralized soda causes excessive loss of water-soluble vitamins.

These vitamins are also water-soluble in body fluids, which means the body cannot store more than the saturation that the tissues and fluids allow. Supply these vitamins daily, and guard against other types of losses.

The food manager who preserves vitamins guards all along the line of selection, storage, and preparation. Keeping foods cool, out of light, in fresh, prime condition, and cooking until just done form the best safeguards.

Vitamin C

It is easy to get enough vitamin C in pleasant ways. In a land of plenty, only ignorance, carelessness, or poverty could prevent an individual or family from having a daily abundance of this vitamin. Four ounces (one-half cup) of a citrus juice, a medium orange, or half a grapefruit will amply supply this vitamin. Also tomatoes or tomato juice (one cup), fresh leafy salads, fresh cabbage, and strawberries are good sources. Probably no other nutrient is packaged more deliciously.

The Four Food Groups specifically provide vitamin C. Neglecting its food sources in the daily diet is inexcusable. Many diets lack vitamin C because people expect a drink—any drink—to function as a real citrus juice.

Vitamin C (ascorbic acid) protects against scurvy, the dread disease of the early voyagers. Their diet of dried meat and hardtack with little other food contained none of this vitamin. Today's diet ideally has enough vitamin C not only to protect against disease but also to give all tissues of the body an abundance of the vitamin. When the diet includes sufficient vitamin C, the tissues are "saturated," or supplied with all they can use.

An abundance of vitamin C aids in keeping the cells intact, helps injured tissues heal more promptly, and helps the tissues resist infection more efficiently.

Adults should have sixty milligrams of vitamin C daily. Although citrus fruit or tomato provides a rule of thumb for dietary inclusion, a number of foods can substitute. Table 5 shows a comparison of servings of various vitamin C foods. The foods supply not only this vitamin but also other factors of nutritional importance. This fact illustrates the great value of getting nutrition from food, since the nutrients we know are packaged together so precisely and cleverly that we should plan our diets in terms of food groups rather than individual nutrients.

The B Vitamins

Again, because nutrients come packaged together, we need consider only three members of the B vitamin group when calculating a diet. When thiamine, riboflavin, and niacin are accounted for in foods, the other B vitamins are present. The B vitamins are also associated with proteins, which the Four Food Groups provide amply.

In general the B vitamins function similarly. They are essential to the effective utilization of the carbohydrates, fats, and proteins by acting mainly as portions of coenzymes that put the energy nutrients promptly through their many processes of oxidation and other changes. The final products of energy metabolism are carbon dioxide (excreted primarily by the lungs), water (excreted by the kidneys, skin, and lungs), and certain nitrogen end products (excreted by the kidneys). The B vitamins tucked into the diet by good food choice provide this efficient utilization of the absorbed simple sugars, fats, amino acids, and minerals.

Lack of the B vitamins has resulted in diseases that have scourged man historically. Beriberi, a disease that causes permanent nerve deterioration, is owing to a lack of thiamine. People who existed mainly on polished, unenriched rice suffered from this disease. Less serious conditions caused by an insufficiency of this vitamin are by no means undamaging to the body. These symptoms appear as indigestion, lack of appetite, constipation, nervousness, and lack of mental alertness. When a combination of these symptoms appears in children, check carefully their thiamine intake.

A disease not known historically by name has been well known by its symptoms—ariboflavinosis. When riboflavin is lacking in the diet, a number of symptoms can appear: skin roughness around the nose and ears; a skin, called "sharkskin," that appears shiny and pulled over the face; persistent sore cracks at the angles of the mouth; and blood vessel changes in the eye. Salve relieves none of these symptoms. Only when each body cell receives the riboflavin needed to get on with the vital business of cell metabolism do the symptoms disappear.

Pellagra, once considered by most doctors an infectious disease, scourged certain Southern States, leaving in its path distress, suffering, and death. In the middle of the second decade of this century Dr. Joseph Goldberger, of the United States Department of Public Health, proved that pellagra resulted from dietary deficiency and that proteins of high biologic value could prevent the disease. Dr. Goldberger did not live to see the B vitamins identified, but thousands in his day benefited from his discovery.

Niacin quite specifically prevents and cures pellagra. Also high biologic proteins when taken in liberal quantities have sufficient of the essential amino acid tryptophan, which the body can convert to niacin. Dr. Goldberger recognized that the pellagrin's diet of refined cornmeal lacked meat and milk. The little protein in cornmeal has less of the essential amino acid tryptophan than most cereals.

Foods provide niacin as the preformed vitamin, or in the case of high biologic proteins as its precursor, tryptophan. Together, leafy green vegetables, whole or enriched cereals, milk, and eggs liberally provide niacin either in the preformed niacin or its precursor. In order to determine the niacin value of a diet, add to the total niacin the niacin produced from the tryptophan in the protein. To quickly estimate, divide the grams of protein in the diet by six, and add the resulting figure to the milligrams of niacin. To illustrate, the calculated choices from the Four Food Groups (page 28) provide 13.1 milligrams of niacin. The 71 grams of protein divided by six gives the figure of 11.8. This 11.8 added to 13.1 milligrams of niacin can be interpreted by this mathematical shortcut as a total of 24.9 milligram equivalents of niacin in the day's food choices.

Vitamin B_{12} is not present in vegetable food except by action of specific microorganisms under controlled conditions. This vitamin, provided in the animal body, is in all flesh food, and also in foods furnished by animals—milk, milk products, and eggs. Some food products have vitamin B_{12} added. The addition of vitamin B_{12} is especially desirable in foods to replace animal-produced foods, such as soy-formula foods used in place of milk. Good food selection easily furnishes the vitamin—for instance, two liberal servings of milk daily and three to four eggs a week.

Vitamin B_{12} deficiency, or an inability to absorb the vitamin, causes a disease of the marrow of the long bones, which make red blood cells. Nerve degeneration and a pernicious type of anemia follow the depletion of this vitamin. Symptoms of the deficiency are much too severe and damaging to risk with careless or experimental self-imposed diets. Children are particularly and relatively quickly damaged by vitamin B_{12} deficiency.

In contrast to vitamin deficiencies, *hypervitaminosis* can occur. Overdose of certain vitamins damages the tissues and cell function, as do vitamin deficiencies. Overdose severe enough to cause toxicity occurs with excessive accumulation of certain fat-soluble vitamins. Such conditions follow excessive overdoses of vitamins A and D either by accidental overdose or by the misapplied idea "If a little is good, more is even better."

Today we commonly hear about "megavitamin therapy." Such therapy involves vitamin doses at least *tenfold* above the recommended daily dietary allowance. The expression is a misnomer, for such therapy is not *vitamin* therapy. In the cells the vitamin is or becomes a coenzyme that attaches to enzymes already existing in the cells. This combination assists in specific metabolic reactions that take place in the body's use of nutrients from food. Such enzyme combinations are necessary, and their functions are completed near or at, the level of the recommended dietary allowances. Each cell contains a fixed amount of vitamin receptor called apoprotein. The vitamin can function only when it has attached to the apoprotein. Vitamins in excess of the optimum amount have to be dealt with as any unnecessary chemical—and usually with side effects, many undesirable.

Let's consider vitamin C (ascorbic acid) as an example. It is essential in preventing scurvy, and it gives tissues a vitally important binding quality. When all vitamin C apoproteins are connected to a vitamin C molecule, the excess vitamin may raise the urine's uric acid level and may cause gout, especially in people who are predisposed to get gout. Also continued use of excessive amounts of vitamin C can depress the activity of vitamin B_{12}.

For medical purposes, megavitamin therapy is sometimes used, for example, to bind a specific poison or to dilate blood vessels. Vitamins used in this way should be considered medicine and should be taken according to a physician's direction and only as long as directed.

On the other hand, megadoses of some vitamins will seriously *damage* vital organs. Vitamin B_6, once thought to be harmless, may cause liver damage. Megadoses of vitamin E have reportedly produced inflammation of the mouth, chapping of the lips, gastrointestinal disturbances, muscle weakness, low blood sugar, increased bleeding, and degenerative changes. It is well established that megadoses of vitamin A cause nerve damage and that megadoses of vitamin D can produce liver toxicity. Certain vitamins in excessive dosages can interfere also with some essential medications, rendering them ineffective.*

Vitamins taken in excess of dietary needs become chemicals that the body must handle as nonnutritional, nonfunctional substances. Damage can follow in their wake. If megavitamins are used as medication they should be prescribed by a physician who monitors the patient's progress to watch for undesirable side effects.

The nutrients—carbohydrates, fats, proteins, minerals, and vitamins—do not function in isolation, but accomplish their work by

---

* V. D. Herbert, *Contemporary Nutrition*, 2:10 (October, 1977).

AN-5

Table 5 Some Food Sources of Several Vitamins

Food	Amount	Vitamin A (IU)	Thiamine mg.	Riboflavin mg.	Niacin mg.	Vitamin C (mg.)
Milk and Milk Products						
Milk, whole	1 cup	350*	.08	.42	.1	2
Cheese, cheddar	1 oz.	350	trace	.12	trace	0
Cheese, cottage, creamed	½ cup	190	.03	.28	.1	0
Yogurt	1 cup	170	.09	.43	.2	2
Eggs						
Eggs	1 egg	590	.05	.15	trace	0
Yolk of egg	1 yolk	580	.04	.07	trace	0
Meat						
Beef, lean	3 oz.	20	.08	.20	5.1	—
Beans and Peas (Legumes), Mature, Nuts						
Almonds	¼ cup	0	.08	.33	1.2	trace
Beans, common varieties, dry, cooked	1 cup	trace	.13	.10	1.5	—
Peanut butter	1 tbsp.	—	.02	.02	2.4	0
Peas, split, dry, cooked	1 cup	100	.37	.22	2.2	—
Vegetables						
Broccoli spears, cooked	1 cup	3,750	.14	.29	1.2	135
Brussels sprouts, cooked	1 cup	680	.10	.18	1.1	113
Cabbage, shredded, raw	1 cup	130	.05	.05	.3	47
Cabbage, cooked	1 cup	220	.07	.07	.5	56
Carrots, diced, cooked	1 cup	15,220	.08	.07	.7	9
Cauliflower, cooked	1 cup	70	.11	.10	.7	66
Greens, various varieties, cooked (spinach as an example)	1 cup	14,580	.13	.25	1.0	50
Peas, green, cooked	1 cup	860	.44	.17	3.7	33

Potatoes, cooked	1 med.	trace	.13	.05	2.0	**22**
Squash, winter, cooked	1 cup	**8,610**	**.10**	**.27**	**1.4**	**27**
Sweet potatoes, baked	1 med.	**8,910**	**.10**	.07	.7	**24**
Tomatoes, cooked	1 cup	**2,180**	**.13**	.07	**1.7**	**40**

Fruits

Apricots, raw	3	**2,890**	.03	.04	.7	10
Cantaloupe, medium	½ melon	**6,540**	.08	.06	**1.2**	**63**
Dates, dry, pitted	1 cup	90	**.16**	**.17**	**3.9**	0
Grapefruit, raw, medium, white	½ fruit	10	.05	.02	.2	**52**
pink or red	½ fruit	**640**	.05	.02	.3	**52**
Orange, raw	1 med.	310	**.16**	.06	.6	**70**
Strawberries, fresh	1 cup	90	.04	.10	**1.0**	**88**

Grain Products

Bread, white, enriched	3 slices	trace	**.18**	**.12**	**1.5**	trace
Bread, whole-wheat	3 slices	trace	**.18**	**.09**	**2.1**	trace
Cornmeal, yellow, enriched	¼ cup	160	**.16**	**.09**	**1.3**	0
Macaroni, cooked	1 cup	0	**.23**	**.14**	**1.9**	0
Oatmeal or rolled oats, cooked	1 cup	0	**.19**	.05	.3	0
Rice, polished, enriched, cooked	1 cup	0	**.19**	.01	**1.6**	0
Wheat, rolled, cooked	1 cup	0	**.17**	.06	**2.1**	0
Wheat germ	¼ cup	0	**.34**	**.12**	.7	0

Fats

Butter	1 tbsp.	**460**	—	—	—	0
Margarine	1 tbsp.	**460**	—	—	—	0

Miscellaneous Items

Yeast, brewer's, dry	1 tbsp.	trace	**1.25**	**.34**	**3.0**	trace

* Bold figures indicate a highly significant vitamin contribution to the diet of one third or more of the recommended allowance for adults per average serving.

a highly developed team approach. The Four Food Groups puzzle makes this "organization" work the best in providing adequate nutrition. A few well-chosen foods each day accomplish the goal of excellent nutrition, and meanwhile the abundant variety of foods available from each puzzle piece not only makes eating an exciting adventure but helps the eater avoid nutritional pitfalls.

Add social graces and good fellowship to proper food selection and preparation, and you foster high morale. This aid to good living accomplishes a happy reaction toward life. At home or at any substitute for the family table—lunch box or eating out—good food furnishing proper nutrition is requisite to life.

Section II

Tailoring According to Need
70/Lifetime Nutrition
83/Engineered Curves
90/Teeth That Last
93/Reducing Health Risks

Chapter 6

LIFETIME NUTRITION

Babies

One of mother's first concerns upon arriving home with her tiny pink angel is feeding it. When? How much? What? Nature answers these questions in a most perfect manner when a healthy mother who is delighted with this specific role breast-feeds her infant. In this instance the food is perfect, and the baby is capable of regulating the timing.

A few years ago doctors sent mother and newborn home on a very strict four-hour schedule, whether baby screamed with hunger after two and a half hours or wanted to sleep peacefully for five hours. Doctors were satisfied; but babies were frustrated, and mothers were exhausted. More recently physicians advise mothers to let baby establish his own schedule, which he will generally do within a few days after arriving home. Baby will often deviate as much as half an hour either side of a set feeding schedule, but do not feed him every time he cries; you soon learn to distinguish between the cry of hunger and the cry of other discomforts.

How can I tell if my baby eats enough? wonder many nursing mothers. The infant probably gets enough to eat if he seems satisfied after about fifteen minutes of eating, if he falls asleep after eating and sleeps for several hours, or if he shows satisfactory weight gain. At birth, baby needs from 360 to 500 calories a day. Human milk and most of the prepared formulas contain twenty calories per ounce, so a newborn baby should take from eighteen to twenty-five ounces a day.

The infant from birth to 1 year of age needs about 0.8 to 1.0 gram of protein per pound of his weight, and fifty calories per pound. A baby weighing twenty pounds, for example, needs about one thousand calories a day and sixteen to twenty grams of protein. For the baby's first three to four months of life, most of these nutritional requirements come from milk—whether it is breast milk, commercially prepared formula, or commercially fortified soy formula.

ABOUT NUTRITION

The infant grows rapidly during his first year. Since each baby is an individual, his rate of development cannot be measured by a precise standard. The average baby doubles his birth weight by 5 months of age, and triples it by 1 year. We can understand such a tremendous weight gain by putting it in terms of adult weight. If an adult gained at such a rate, a 125-pound person would weigh 250 pounds in five months and tip the scales at 375 pounds after 12 months. No wonder infant nutrition is so important!

"Hey! What's that lumpy stuff Mom's stuck in my mouth? I'm going to gag!" Junior may react to his first solid food.

Twenty years have seen many controversial theories regarding when to start solid foods. A few years ago cereals, fruit, and vegetables were not introduced until the child reached 12 to 18 months; but now the pendulum has swung over to the point where mothers brag about the quantity of cereal their 2½-week-old consumes. After weighing the advantages and disadvantages, most nutritionists agree that some babies may need and can accept solids at about 2½ to 3 months of age. But breast-fed infants may not need solids until they reach 6 months. The development and appetite of a baby, rather than chronological age, should determine when you add solid foods. Every new addition of solid food should be in approximately half-teaspoon-sized servings.

Cereals are usually the first solid food given. Enriched cereals supplement baby's iron-poor milk diet. A normal full-term infant does not require earlier additions of iron, because at birth the child's liver reserves iron to tide him over the all-milk period of his life. Orange juice and pureed fruit and vegetables may follow soon after cereal, with hard-boiled egg yolks, custards, and cottage cheese added after 6 months. Baby should eat bland food with very little additional salt or sweetener. Adults may enjoy condiments and spices, but they should not use them for seasoning baby's food.

Babies on a vegetarian diet can start on protein foods such as pureed cottage cheese (plain or with fruit), egg yolk (pureed with water or milk), high protein cereals with milk, and plain yogurt. When the baby becomes able to eat coarse foods, legumes (dried peas or beans) may be added along with peanut butter, whole-grain cereals, very soft meat analogs (commercially prepared vegetable protein), and tofu (soybean curd).

Some vegetarian protein foods do not contain as much iron as does meat. Therefore, each day the vegetarian baby needs to eat some foods high in iron, such as iron-fortified cereal, egg yolk, legumes, dark-green vegetables, or meat analog with whole grains. (Adapted from *Feeding the Vegetarian Infant,* 1978.)

Many parents do not realize that even infants need water. Acquaint baby with the taste of water during his first few months so that it will be a regular part of his diet now, and for the rest of his life. Older children may not care for water if they established their eating habits before mother regularly introduced water. Boil water and and cool it to room temperature for the infant's bottle, and offer water in a cup several times a day to the toddler. Always offer the water without hurry and without concern; if the child refuses it, just offer it again a little later.

A baby accepts new foods best when he is hungry and not overly tired. They should be introduced one at a time in tiny amounts, accompanied by some of his favorite foods. The young baby is not adept at carrying solid food from the front to the back of the mouth. Therefore, place only half spoonfuls well back on the tongue with the baby semireclined, until he improves his swallowing skills. Give him several days to adjust to one new food before you add another. Do not force a baby to eat a food he does not care for; instead, an item he refuses should not appear on the menu again for a few days. If he still refuses the food, substitute a food equal in nutritional value and offer the rejected food again a month or so later. A baby will quickly sense others' dislike for food he eats.

Keep rich desserts and pastry to a minimum so that the child does not early acquire a taste for sweets to the exclusion of other foods. Feed baby foods varying in both taste and texture toward the end of the first year. The child accustomed to many kinds of foods will less likely be a finicky eater.

Wean from the bottle to a cup during the latter part of the first year. At about 5 months, baby should discover how to drink from a cup. By 9 months, offer milk in a cup instead of one of his regular feedings. Then gradually replace all breast or bottle feedings by the cup, although the morning and bedtime bottles may continue for some time. Nursing mothers discover that a gradual weaning, placing less and less demands on the mammary glands, slows the flow of milk and minimizes discomfort, and baby will rarely experience any physical discomfort or emotional trauma during a gradual transition to cow's milk from breast or formula feeding. The 2-year-old who takes several bottles or breast feedings a day may become anemic as a result of exclusion of solid foods containing essential vitamins and minerals.

Toddler

Sometime during the second year, when a child can pick up objects between the thumb and index finger, he will try feeding himself, much to a tidy mother's dismay. For the next few months, temporarily abandon table manners as the child explores the texture of his food and develops his own dexterity. Although you need not tolerate playing with food, baby enjoys feeling his oatmeal and testing its possibilities. As he begins to master a spoon his mother may gently encourage a few social graces, keeping in mind that she should not meet the inevitable accidents with disapproval or scolding.

The second year, the child's growth rate slows, and he enters the "terrible twos." Suddenly a normal, hearty eater picks at his food or even rejects entire meals. Parents must keep calm, for a healthy, active child *will* eat when he is hungry, since he can probably judge the amounts (but not kinds) of food he needs better than his parents. Since his growth rate has decreased, so has his appetite.

This period triggers many problem eaters. Junior refuses to eat; his mother panics! She bribes him with toys and desserts; he whines. She threatens spankings and early bedtime; he clamps his lips and kicks his high chair. She tries "one bite for Grandpa and one bite for teddy bear"; and he spits.

Mother thinks, He'll get sick if he doesn't eat.

Junior thinks, This is great! I'll try it again tomorrow. And so the long battle begins.

What should a mother do? If she presents nourishing, attractive food in easy-to-handle forms at regular intervals with no appetite-dulling snacks between times, the healthy, active toddler will eat all he needs. If he refuses a meal, excuse him without a fuss, not to eat again until he is ready for a meal. The child given an unnecessary amount of parental supervision and vigilance usually develops into a problem eater. Orphanages and large families have very few picky eaters because they have no time for individual pampering.

Serve the variety of foods in the Four Food Groups in *small portions* to the toddler. The total daily intake recommended is as follows:

Fruit and Vegetable Group .... 4 servings
> Include at least 4 ounces of orange juice or other vitamin C-rich food.
> Portions of other foods may be 2 to 3 tablespoonfuls.
> Include a dark-green or -yellow vegetable daily.

Cereal and Bread Group .... 4 servings
> Half slices of bread and 2 or 3 level tablespoon portions of cereal may count as servings for children.

Protein Group .... 2 servings
    Include an egg 3 or 4 times a week.
    Give other high Protein foods once or twice a day in 2 to 3
       tablespoon amounts.
Milk Group
    Three cups or more may be given if not displacing other foods.
       The child may take less or very small amounts of milk for
       short periods of time without harm.

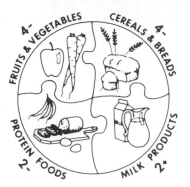

    Better to serve small portions and then repeat as desired rather than start with a discouragingly large portion of food. Follow this rule: one tablespoon (standard measuring type) of food for each year of age. The toddler may need five or six regularly scheduled feedings a day rather than three large meals. He will more easily eat and better tolerate soft foods simply prepared. Avoid skins and seeds of fruits, rich sauces, and fried foods.

Preschool Children

    Preschoolers are delightful, busy creatures. Mother, who waited eagerly for baby to walk, now wishes he would occasionally stop running. The preschooler finds many new and wonderful things to explore—including food.
    The preschooler usually prefers plain food—no gravies, sauces, spices, and very few mixtures. Preschool children generally prefer mild-flavored foods, because of high sensitivity to taste; they find rich, spicy foods strong and distasteful. They frequently prefer raw vegetables. The child's ability to chew should somewhat determine the texture of his food.
    Capitalize upon chewing as a new venture to the young one with new teeth. The youngster will relish crispy carrots, crunchy

zwieback, juicy apple or pear slices, and refreshing lettuce wedges. Finger foods rate high. A child may refuse certain foods because they are clumsy to manage at the end of a spoon, and not because of their taste. A large spear of broccoli may appear forbidding to small chubby fingers, whereas he can easily pick up one or two small broccoli buds to explore. He may tire of eating cereal with a spoon, but he will thrill if it is thick and offered to him as finger-food balls.

Desire for food may be erratic for the preschooler, so an occasional "won't eat" phase should not cause undue concern. A healthy child eventually gets hungry and eats satisfactorily over a period of time. On the other hand, food jags frequent the preschool years. If Johnny decides he will exist on peanut butter sandwiches and celery sticks for a day or two, it is no disaster. Accept the food jags instead of blowing them out of proportion, and he will abandon them in due time. If, however, a jag of foods of low nutrient density seems to persist, it might be good to try running out of the foods, making no effort to replace them. Parents, instead of putting too much emphasis on eating, should establish mealtime as a happy, relaxed family occasion.

A child tends to dawdle at this age. Fortunately, he does not have the adult sense of time and does not feel rushed. Urging him to "hurry" may spoil his pleasure in life and in eating. Why not let the child begin his meal before the rest of the family sits down so that you need not rush him? A child served small portions or allowed to serve himself may do a better job of eating everything on his plate. Making a "clean plate" a familiar rule may lead to a habit of overeating, which can carry over into later life and lead to overweight. Many mothers wonder whether to allow a child to eat dessert who leaves food on his plate. If dessert is an occasional treat, as it should be, the problem solves itself. As a rule, a fair consumption of food served on the plate justifies at least a small serving of dessert eaten with the rest of the family. Far better to set a good example in eating for Junior to follow than to nag.

Active children may become overtired and, although excessively hungry, cannot eat properly. Proper rest and a sensible eating schedule governed by the child's needs may correct this. Many pre-schoolers snack on candy, soft drinks, chips, and other low nutrient density foods virtually all day. When they are big enough to help themselves to these foods, parents complain "I cannot do anything about it!" The answer may be simple. Seldom have candy, chips, or soft drinks in the house because they tempt children and adults alike. Instead, a wise parent furnishes nutritious food possibilities, such as fresh carrot and celery strips, fresh fruit, whole-grain breads and crackers, and unsweetened cereals.

Recent trends indicate a movement away from established family meal times toward constant eating called "grazing." This trend can and has led to many nutritional problems predominately in consumption of high fat, high calorie foods containing few vitamins, minerals, and fiber. If between-meal eating is allowed, serve foods light enough not to spoil the appetite for the next meal, and make them contribute to the child's nutritional need. Such foods may be fruit juice, fat-modified milk and milk products, dry whole-grained cereal, or whole grained-crackers and bread.

Chubby, dimpled 5-year-olds delight parents and photographers but worry nutritionists. Most normal 4- to 5-year-olds are thin and gangly. The cute, plump 5-year-old often matures into the obese adult who battles overweight for a lifetime. This amplifies the significance of utilizing the Four Food Groups puzzle, emphasizing more fruits and vegetables and less sweets, desserts, empty-calorie snacks, and excess low-nutrient, starchy foods.

School-age Children

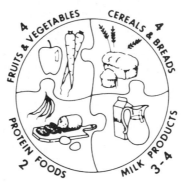

Play activities easily divert eager, happy-go-lucky grade school youngsters from eating. Without vigilant mothers, "Little Leaguers" grab a slice of bread and peanut butter and race off to the ball field. If schools did not require students to remain in their seats or in the cafeteria for at least fifteen minutes during noon hour, most children would skip lunch in favor of play.

In general, the school-age child copies the eating habits of those about him. If teacher has chocolate-marshmallow cookies every day for lunch, then "Little Miss" must eat chocolate-marshmallow cookies every day for lunch. The child compares home eating habits with the eating habits of his peers, thus discovering that the world encompasses much more than his small family circle. Group influence is important, and the child explores new foods his friends introduce and may reject some of his old favorites that his playmates do not accept. Fortunately the schoolchild has a strong incentive to "grow big and strong" like his parents, older siblings, or favorite sports star.

Schedule meals around school hours. Occasionally, working mothers may serve hasty, skimpy breakfasts or no breakfast at all, which not only sends children off to school without proper energy and vitality for the day, but also paves the way for them to become adults who just aren't hungry for breakfast. Avoid a very rushed schedule or undue excitement as much as possible, because disturbances dull a child's appetite.

Schoolrooms are great breeding grounds for communicable diseases. These illnesses usually decrease the appetite, while increasing the child's nutritional needs to compensate for fever and infection. Hence, mother's ingenuity plays a decisive role as she turns an everyday salad into a clown's face, or a plain custard into a pleasant surprise by adding bits of bright-colored fruit. Necessary fruit juices go down much better with a flexible drinking straw.

The school-age child can eat almost anything an adult eats. Allow him a certain freedom of choice, however. Since most children arrive home from school "starved," supper hour should be set to take this into consideration. If an after school snack is chosen, advanced planning can insure the availability of such nutritious foods as oatmeal cookies and fat modified milk, fresh fruit that has been washed and prepared for eating, or yogurt and fruit.

Weight problems, either overweight or underweight, may predominate in the school-age child. The inactive child who nibbles all day long often grows overweight. Unfortunately the obese child tends to become the adult who battles the weight problem all his life. On the other hand, the nervous child may lose interest in food and subsequently lose weight. He then has no padding for his falls and more readily succumbs to illness.

Both problems need the cooperation of the parents. Encourage the nibbling child to limit his munching to regularly scheduled meals and emphasize vegetables and fruits and de-emphasize sweets, snack foods, and high-fat foods. Encourage him to participate in outdoor activities and make the television set less prominent in family life.

The underweight child may need supplemental feedings of milk drinks and other high-calorie foods to help him gain weight. Overemphasis on table manners may adversely affect the child's appetite. With a few exceptions the lacto-ovo-vegetarian child will follow the same food guide as the meat-eating child.

Fruit and Vegetable Group .... 4 servings*
  2 servings of which supply vitamin C
    (citrus, tomatoes, cabbage, strawberries)
  1 serving of which supplies vitamin A
    (a dark-green or deep-yellow vegetable)
Cereal and Bread Group .... 4 servings*
  At least 2 servings of whole grains
Protein Group .... 2 servings*
  Includes legumes (mature beans and peas), eggs, wheat
    protein foods, soy protein foods, nuts, and nut butters
Milk Group .... 3-4 servings

Teens

One day, after parents have stored away the high chairs and training bikes, they suddenly come face to face with a bewildering creation—a teenager. The teenager of 13 is mostly child, and then with varying stages of changes through the next few years, at 19 he is mostly adult.

Teen years bring the second rapid growth spurt, which girls usually reach at ages 12 to 14 and boys at ages 14 to 16. Mothers who once begged and bribed a small boy to eat stand aghast as that same boy, now in his teens, eats three peanut-butter-and-jam sandwiches, two apples, four cookies, and a quart of milk, and then asks, "What's for dinner?" Not only do their bodies grow at an alarming rate, but they also undergo the stress and nervous strain of developing their personalities. They strive for independence. This accumulation of growth presents a nutritional challenge to meet the expanding needs of the young adult. While caloric needs soar and the other nutritional needs increase, the untrained teenage appetite, unfortunately, does not always crave nutritionally adequate food.

Dr. Alice Garrett Marsh describes this period as a time when practically all teenagers tend to have a few food peculiarities that are their right. Mixtures and casseroles aren't favorites; they usually

---

* The servings sizes in these Four Food Groups can vary from a scant tablespoon to nearly half a cup.

prefer their foods separate. They like some informal meals to which they can come and go—especially when working on a special project. Food and eating are preferred with little fanfare.

Teen years give the young person a last chance for excellent body building. Boys, interested in muscle and body building, should consciously consider the rewards of balanced meals. However, their appetites know no bounds, and they will eat almost anything and everything they can get their hands on, including low-nutrient-density foods such as candy bars, cake, soft drinks, and shakes. Wise mothers provide generous servings from fruit, vegetables, whole-grains, milk, and vegetable protein foods to satisfy hunger and provide strong, vibrant bodies for their teen boys.

Teenage girls are the most poorly fed of all age groups. Their greatest deficiencies are calcium and iron, since they most often exclude from their diet milk, eggs, vegetables (including potatoes), and bread. The young lady, extremely weight and figure conscious, experiments with any fad diet, diet pill, and noncaloric food or beverage. Her eating habits fluctuate—one day indulging in French pastries and chocolate creams, and the next day eating only grapefruit and hard-boiled eggs so that she can squeeze into a new dress one and a half sizes too small. Her drive toward independence and her need to break away from family food patterns exceed her teenage brother's. Her mind whirls with thoughts of dating, fashionable clothes, and popularity rather than the beautiful woman nature intended her to be, capable of bearing healthy, vigorous babies at some future time.

Skin problems may erupt during the teen years. A well-balanced diet emphasizing fruits, vegetables (especially green and yellow), whole grains, milk, and sufficient water to help remove wastes is the best dietary defense. Some foods, such as rich desserts, fats, chocolate, and nuts, seem to trigger acne.

Overweight may become a problem for young adults who limit their exercise to lying before the television or talking on the telephone for hours. Instead of carefully planning their caloric intake to match their growth and activity, the teenager's concept of weight control often consists of skipping meals (especially breakfast), omitting bread, milk, potatoes, and other vegetables, because they are "too fattening," then, ironically, snacking on soft drinks, candy, chips, and sweets. The breakfast skipper usually encounters a midmorning slump, thus reducing activity. A sweet snack may give a temporary lift, but it dulls the appetite for lunch and wears off just in time to necessitate after-school munching. A large, late dinner tops off the day, and several bedtime snacks follow. Consequently the overweight teen feels he gains weight even though he "hardly eats anything."

Dr. Marsh says that a food is a poor choice unless it satisfies needs other than hunger. It should furnish protein, minerals, and/or vitamins—which soda pop, candy, or syrupy things don't have. Rich desserts supply calories in abundance, but the other nutrients, though present, are very low. The wise teen will choose from real fruit or vegetable juices, milk drinks that are not overrich, crisp raw vegetables, and sandwiches made with good-quality bread and nourishing fillings. These foods—not sweet rolls or doughnuts or pop—build healthy bodies.

The vegetarian teenager may worry that his food choices in restaurants and fast-food places will be severely limited. While it is true that he will have to be selective, experience has shown that the lacto-ovo-vegetarian can find a variety of good foods to eat away from home. Chinese, Mexican, and spaghetti-type restaurants often have many no-meat items already on the menu. When choosing from any menu, ask which items contain meat and which items could be served without meat. Most restaurants have a vegetable plate that they will make up upon request, consisting of the vegetables for the day, usually including a potato and sometimes macaroni and cheese, or cottage or yellow cheese. Other possibilities are pancakes, pizza, hero or submarine sandwiches without the cold cuts, fruit plates, and salad bars, and cafeteria-style restaurants. Listed among the appetizers of many restaurants are such vegetarian items as French onion soup (ask whether it includes bacon), fruit cocktail, vegetable or fruit juices, cottage cheese, and sherbet. An appetizer of this nature with a potato, another vegetable, and bread makes a good meal.

Merely asking whether a menu item is "vegetarian" or stating that you "want no meat" may not give the waitress sufficient information. State that you do not want any meat, fish, or poultry, including meat stocks, and then ask about the menu items. Most waitresses do not consider fish as meat, nor do they realize that you do not want bacon on your salad or green beans unless you state thus.

So, go ahead. Go out and eat with the gang occasionally. Ask the hamburger place whether they will make you a hamburger with everything but the hamburger. Many places will. Order a grilled-cheese sandwich and a salad along with a tall glass of milk. Take your cheese pizza with olives or mushrooms. Or suggest going to an Italian restaurant, and ask that your dishes be made with plain tomato sauce without the meat.

ABOUT NUTRITION

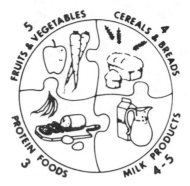

   The Four Food Groups furnish the best eating pattern for teens. The servings of food recommended each day for teenagers are as follows:

Fruit and Vegetable Group .... 5 servings
    2 servings of which supply vitamin C
      (citrus, tomatoes, cabbage, strawberries, etc.)
    1 serving of which supplies vitamin A
      (dark-green or deep-yellow vegetable)
Cereal and Bread Group .... 4 servings
    At least 2 servings of whole grains
Protein Group .... 3 servings
Milk Group .... 4-5 servings
    For weight watchers, low-fat milk

   Again, Dr. Marsh advises parents to have a special part in teen-age nutrition. In spite of the size of shoes, the sophistication of the clothes, the adult richness of a son's voice, the grown-up beauty of a daughter, the ability of both to do things, it is the parents' work to supply the food, prepare it, and serve it in a good home climate.

   This does not mean that teens should not take on responsibilities of many sorts. They can earn money, take on more home responsibilities, cook, clean, garden, farm, build, care for younger children. However, if the teenager takes the responsibility of getting a good profession or trade, he or she must do so during the teen and young adult years.

   The responsibility of food, three times a day, seven days a week, should rest on the parents, Dr. Marsh maintains. Good nutritional advantages of the home and a creative home atmosphere are mainly

AN-6

the work of the parents. Teens are not ready for such total responsibility. They are ready to become "officers of the day," first assistants and strong support to parents, but not to take on parents' responsibilities. With parents fully responsible and on the job in the fuller sense of homemaking, the teenager can be free to carry increasing responsibilities that prepare him for life. In the meantime, he can feel the support he needs as he readies himself in education and daily experiences for a highly competitive world.

Best of all, those who have experienced good parental support during the teen years and into young adulthood have, in turn, a priceless preparation for their responsibility to their children. The children of today's successful family are tomorrow's parents with an "inherited" blueprint for establishing another successful home.

Chapter 7

ENGINEERED CURVES

Americans have a weighty problem. On the one hand, our society demands that we appear slim, bordering on emaciation; and on the other hand, the media scream that food and fun are synonymous. Grocery store tabloids and magazines headline the "latest" way to lose ugly fat, yet high-calorie food is temptingly accessible everywhere. Vending machines, convenience food stores with extended hours, and the proliferation of restaurants and fast-food eateries persuade us that we are almost always hungry. Skinny TV stars, tall, lithe models, and the "thin executive" image demand that overweight people cannot be accepted and successful. And so being on a "diet" is the thing for everyone to do—old, young, male, female.

Why is nearly 30 percent of America's population overweight? Social activities encourage the eating of high-calorie desserts and snacks. After a person reaches 25 years of age, body processes tend to slow down. Similarly, physical activity usually diminishes as the person can afford more laborsaving devices for the home, such as a riding mower, automatic garage-door opener, and electric can opener; as he advances in his job from manual and active labor to a more sedentary phase; and as he uses escalators, elevators, motorized golf carts, et cetera. Many people unwittingly try to compensate for emotional problems or stress by the comfort of eating. Structured eating, such as family meals, has been largely replaced by individuals' eating whatever is handy whenever they feel like it.

The persons who stop smoking may notice a particular problem with weight gain. Smoking dulls the senses of taste and smell, and former smokers suddenly discover the delicious flavors of food they have not really tasted since they began to smoke. In addition, they have the almost uncontrollable physical habit of reaching for something to put in their mouth.

Overweight people encounter a variety of complex problems. They have a much greater chance of developing a chronic illness such as high blood pressure, heart disease, arthritis, diabetes, or liver and gallbladder disturbances. Emotionally they probably feel dissatisfied with their body image. They may forfeit certain positions of employment because of their appearance and limited activity. Overweight people are usually annoyed to find that the smartest fashions are in small sizes. And many forms of public transportation are extremely difficult for the very portly to use.

Lacto-ovo-vegetarians have a dietary advantage over their meat-eating counterparts. Most lacto-ovo-vegetarian diets contain less fat and therefore have fewer calories, because of the absence of meat fat. They also include larger amounts of fiber, because of the increased consumption of fruit and vegetables. A low-fat, high-fiber diet is a positive step in reducing calories.

The first step in reducing body weight is to visit a physician. He can determine the probable cause of weight gain and any physical problem or complication involved, and he can suggest accurate weight reduction resources. The philosophy of adequate weight reduction is to make lifelong changes in eating and exercise patterns. Although crash diets may reduce weight temporarily, at best they may upset nutritional well-being, and at worst they can damage health for life.

Before successfully mastering overweight, a person needs to understand the causes of his weight problem. Realizing why a person rewards himself with desserts and doughnuts, why he is constantly nibbling on chocolates and chips, and what role food plays in his life greatly simplifies setting the stage for a lifestyle change. Perhaps the only problem is the person's inactivity. Or it may be as simple as not realizing how often and how much he eats.

The individual should determine the desirable weight for his age, sex, height, and activity. He should weigh himself weekly, keeping an accurate record of weight fluctuations. Body weight normally fluctuates a little from day to day, because of fluid retention or loss. Even those who do not need to lose weight should consult the scales regularly to watch for sudden, unaccountable weight loss, which may be the first indication of illness. Normal-weight people should guard against gaining more than five pounds above desirable weight.

A wise reduction diet maintains the nutrition of the individual while reducing his weight. It consists of a reasonable variety of ordinary, palatable low-calorie foods. Foods like whole grains, fruit, and vegetables contain bulk to give a feeling of fullness, but they are moderate to low in calories. Choosing a moderate to low-calorie diet can be extremely simple. For one day, almost any choice of foods from the Four Food Groups, in the recommended number of adult servings, adds up to only 1,100 to 1,200 calories, with needed nutrients in good supply. (See page 24 for sample menu.) Most moderately active adults can lose weight on 1,200 calories a day.

Many overweight people do not eat "meals." Instead they are continually verbalizing, "I'm on a diet, so I'm skipping lunch [or breakfast or dinner]," while they consume thousands of calories a day with a little bite here and a little bite there. Typically, these individuals feel they hardly eat a thing, and yet their intake might look like this:

	Calories
MORNING	
2 cups coffee, cream/sugar	130
2 Danish (one gobbled, one nibbled later)	400
1 praline	300
NOON	
1 cup cream-style soup	200
6 saltines	100
1 cup coffee, cream/sugar	65
MIDAFTERNOON	
1 roll Life Savers	100
1 diet soft drink	1
3 handfuls potato chips with sour-cream dip	300
DINNER	
1 Salad	20
3 tablespoons Roquefort dressing	375
BEFORE BED	
1 cup ice cream (licked from container)	150
1 sliver chocolate cake, extra dab of frosting, lots of extra crumbs	200
	2,341

Slow eating and thorough chewing may aid in losing weight, for they reduce the speed of consumption and allows a person to be aware of what he is eating. However, lingering around food after an eating session can encourage second, third, or fourth servings of tempting food. Too much variety of food at one session may invite excessive intake. Tense conversations or watching entertainment on television while eating may encourage rapid and/or unconscious eating. To be in control of eating, we must deliberately and thoughtfully choose what we eat.

Sometimes we neglect the importance of coordinated exercise when we want to adopt a new lifestyle. Though calorie expenditure by specific exercise may not seem striking, regular moderate exercise benefits all age groups, especially the middle-aged and older. Such a program usually allows a person to eat a variety of food, including an occasional dessert. Exercise improves muscle tone, stimulates circulation, gives a sense of well-being, and provides a release for stress that could lead to excessive eating or other harmful side effects. Walking, though a lost art, is one of the best exercises, since it involves many muscles, and since when done briskly it improves cardiovascular fitness.

Exercise is often underrated as a means of burning calories. True, one must burn up 3,500 calories to burn up the equivalent of one pound of fat. But a close look at what small, consistent changes are necessary to do this reaffirms the benefits of regular exercise.

It takes only about seven calories of energy (three minutes) for the average person to remove three loads of laundry from a washer and place them into a dryer, adjust the dial, and remove the clothes from the dryer when dry. However, it takes the average person approximately 64.3 calories to unload three loads of laundry from the washer (1.5 minutes), make three round-trips to the clothesline (three minutes of walking), hang up the laundry (ten minutes), and make another round-trip to the clothesline when the clothes are dry (one minute) to take them down (three minutes). So, if you were to hang three loads of laundry out on the line once a week for a month, you would burn 257.2 calories instead of the twenty-eight calories you would burn up by using an automatic dryer. Or, looking at it another way, in 52 weeks you would burn up enough *more* calories to remove .82 of a pound of fat!

The difference between riding a power lawn mower one hour (130 calories) and pushing a power lawn mower one hour (240 calories) is 110 calories. In two months (nine weeks) of pushing the lawn mower one hour a week insted of riding a mower, you would expend 990 more calories, or burn .28 of a pound of fat. Therefore, in two months (nine weeks) of pushing the lawn mower instead of hiring the neighbor boy to do it, you would burn 2,160 calories, or .6 pound of fat.

Climbing one flight of stairs burns 3.5 calories (thirty seconds), while riding an elevator up one flight burns .3 calories and takes about fifteen seconds. If you went up these stairs five times a day and five days a week for one year, you would use 4,550 calories walking (only 390 riding). The difference could mean getting rid of 1.19 pounds a year while adding only six extra minutes a week to your schedule.

Those who wish to reduce can usually eat regular foods from the grocery store or restaurant if they follow these tips:

- Schedule small regular meals.
- Take only moderate servings and avoid seconds.
- Reduce or eliminate late night eating.
- Reduce all sweets and desserts.
- Make tempting unnecessary foods as inaccessible as possible.
- Plan satisfying hobbies or activities that will emotionally replace food as a reward.
- Welcome opportunities to exercise.

Motivation forms an essential part of successful weight reduction. Some people find that striving for a reasonable goal in a specified length of time spurs them on to success. Group encouragement stimulates some, and weight charts help others. Placing a red check on the calendar each day you hold to your food and exercise resolutions may add incentive. Employ whatever motivates you to lose weight sensibly. Say these words aloud to yourself three times every day, "I choose to lose."

Underweight individuals may battle just as hard to attain a desirable weight as do overweight persons. For them also, correction of body weight depends on motivation and knowledge of food values. Many a parent mistakenly urges a thin child to eat anything he wants and anytime he wants, to encourage weight gain. Usually this establishes a lifestyle that the child as an adult will find a great detriment.

Do not envy thin people. The underweight have less resistance to infection and experience more fatigue. Underweight during pregnancy increases the likelihood of complications. Adipose tissue is desirable in the right amount for padding, for keeping the body warm, and as a supporting energy store in time of food deprivation. Poor nutrition and underweight are often closely related.

It is a paradox of our times that while the majority of women in our society need to lose, anorexia nervosa is becoming more prevalent. Anorexia nervosa is a condition seen mostly in young women. The afflicted have such a strong fear of becoming fat that they literally starve themselves. Some die. Bulimia, on the other hand, is a gorge-purge syndrome in which the bulimic stuffs himself with food, then either induces vomiting or takes laxatives to rid himself of the unwanted calories. Both conditions require careful and professional physical and emotional evaluations.

The physician should determine the cause of underweight. It occurs most frequently and is most serious in youth, when the young body needs ample supplies of energy, protein, vitamins, and minerals. The underweight person is often tense and nervous, owing in part to poor nutrition. Often he eats irregularly, selects poor foods, and has either a spasmodic or indifferent appetite. He may not receive adequate rest, which makes him more tense and nervous. Unfortunately, the underweight person often considers himself to have good health because he is thin. Thinness and wellness are not synonymous.

Underweight individuals often mistakenly believe that they eat a well-balanced diet, just because they are thin. Therefore, the first dietary suggestion for underweight people is to determine what they eat and revise this if necessary to follow the Four Food Groups and the Dietary Guidelines. Next, they should ascertain their desirable weight and keep accurate records of weight gains. Then, they should increase in small amounts the calories consumed daily by adding high-calorie and calorie-dense foods to the diet. Calorie-dense foods include sauces, gravies, margarine, oil, peanut butter, and smaller amounts of jam, jelly, syrup, honey, molasses, et cetera. The increase in the amount of food eaten should begin gradually, because a sudden overload of food may result in loss of appetite.

Rapid weight gains usually increase adipose tissue only, instead of coordinated gains of muscle, body protein, and body fat. A weight gain of two pounds a week is a reasonable goal. To facilitate this gain, add four hundred to eight hundred calories a day above the amount needed to maintain body weight.

Regularly scheduled meals and snacks prepared attractively and appealingly and eaten in an unhurried, pleasant atmosphere will stimulate lagging appetites. Correct eating patterns coupled with regular exercise stimulate circulation, build muscle tone, and often alleviate the underweight problem. It is erroneous to assume that all thin people are physically fit. Indeed, many thin people are dreadfully physically unfit. Adequate rest and periodic relaxation lend a calm to the spirit and decrease the calories expended for nervous energy.

Maintaining desirable weight, being neither overweight nor underweight, is good and inexpensive life insurance. People can correct improper weight by adjusting eating patterns to either decrease or increase calories while still maintaining high levels of necessary nutrients. Ideally, such a program of positive health begins during childhood with well-balanced meals, regular exercise, and adequate rest and recreation. The wise family will schedule activities around such essentials. By weighing yourself regularly, you can discover weight discrepancies early and alter them immediately while the problem is relatively simple and most easily corrected.

Chapter 8

TEETH THAT LAST

A person does not have pearly white teeth, beautiful and free of fillings, as a matter of chance. They directly result from heredity, good nutrition, and daily care. Teeth break food into small particles that digestive juices and enzymes can act upon. Unless solid foods are chewed and mixed with saliva, the body cannot properly digest them or utilize the nutrients. The digestion of starches begins in the mouth when saliva mixes with food during the chewing process.

One of the most prevalent diseases among humans is dental caries, affecting an estimated 90 percent of the world's population. Children are highly susceptible, especially after deciduous teeth erupt. Dental plaque, a transparent gelatinous material filled with bacteria, is a precursor of caries. Plaque traps bacteria, and they use the carbohydrates in the food passing through the mouth to form organic acids. These acids dissolve the enamel and can progress to the dentin and even into the dental pulp, which houses the nerve.

The foundation, or basic structure, of the teeth to a great extent determines their wearability. Properly formed teeth containing adequate nutrients resist decay. Tooth and bone structures begin growing about the seventh week of intrauterine life and necessitate that pregnant women ingest generous supplies of protein, calcium, phosphorus, and vitamins A and D. Nutritional conditions prevailing during tooth formation, both before and after birth, affect tooth structure most.

That fluoridation of water helps reduce dental caries by about 50 percent has been long known. More recently, studies have shown that one milligram of fluoride a day taken during pregnancy can dramatically improve the development, strength, and whiteness of the baby's teeth. It can virtually ensure that the teeth will remain carie-free through most of childhood. Fluoridated water cannot provide enough fluoride, so pregnant women should take one 2.2-milligram sodium fluoride tablet daily. Best results occur if they take it either on an empty stomach or without milk, milk products, or antacids. These substances interfere with fluoride absorption.

The infant at birth, although seemingly toothless, has nearly all of his deciduous teeth and several of his permanent teeth partly developed, and therefore requires continued supplies of protein, calcium, and phosphorus found in milk. By the third month you should fortify baby's milk diet with vitamins A and D to ensure healthy gums and teeth. According to the discretion of the physician, accomplish this supplementation by food additions or supplements of suitable quantity.

Calcium and phosphorus are the chief mineral components of teeth, and vitamins A, C, and D regulate the building processes of these particular tissues. Even after the teeth form, adequate supplies of calcium and phosphorus help prevent dental caries. During enamel formation and calcification, the daily ingestion of minute quantities of fluoride, taken either in fluoridated water or in supplemental drops or pills, makes the enamel decay resistant throughout life. Topical application of fluoride gives further protection. The results of fluoride intake are most effective when fluoride ingestion is begun before the tooth buds erupt.

The inclusion of certain foods in the daily menu assures adequate amounts of the essential building materials. Milk supplies three of the nutrients needed for lasting teeth: protein, calcium, and phosphorus. Fortified milk furnishes vitamin D. Some vitamin C-rich foods are citrus fruits, strawberries, and raw cabbage. Since not all people have the benefit of fluoridated water, a dentist or physician may prescribe fluorine in pill or liquid form. With the exception of fluorine, the simple Four Food Groups provide all nutrients necessary to ensure decay-resistant teeth. In certain spots on this earth there is just the right amount of fluoride salt occurring naturally in the drinking water. No additional fluorine is needed.

Preserving teeth requires not only eating the right nutrients but also including the right food textures in the diet. If you expect your teeth to last, put them to good use. Even during infancy the sucking action aids jaw development. Later, chewing develops and maintains strong teeth and jaws and healthy gums. The average diet consists of two types of food textures: *detergent foods,* which sweep over, around, and between teeth and soft tissues; and *impacting foods,* which are soft and sticky, require little chewing, and adhere to the teeth. Apples, raw carrots, whole-wheat bread, and hard crusts are detergent foods. Mashed potatoes, white bread, jam, stewed prunes, and ice cream exemplify impacting foods. The average diet today contains too many soft foods to maintain healthy gums and teeth.

Why not end each meal with a detergent food, then brush the teeth thoroughly? If you cannot brush after every meal, swish water between your teeth to remove much of the food and bacteria that otherwise adhere.

Dental caries are infections carried by cariogenic streptococci that act upon specific carbohydrates. Sucrose—found in a concentrated form in table sugar—is the most highly cariogenic carbohydrate. Among the less cariogenic sugars are lactose (milk sugar), fructose, glucose, and sorbitol.

One important factor affecting the production of dental caries is the frequency of sugar intake. Once the sugar has saturated the plaque, acid producing begins immediately. This acid condition remains for twenty to thirty minutes, and the mineral enamel begins to dissolve. If a sweet is eaten promptly and the teeth brushed or the mouth rinsed very soon after eating, minimal harm will occur. But if the sweet is nibbled often over an extended period of time, great harm will take place. Sugar-sweetened soft drinks, which are not recommended for other reasons, are not as potentially dangerous as sticky sweet foods that adhere to the teeth. However, several soft drinks between meals or one drink sipped over a long period is harmful. Sugar eaten with a meal is less harmful, because of the increased salivary flow, which buffers the acid-producing process and washes away food particles.

Especially in children's mouths, the cariogenic streptococci grow easily and rapidly. Therefore, it is of prime importance to a child's dental health to limit the sucrose-containing foods in the diet—sticky sweets between meals, in particular. If snacks do form part of the diet, choose them from the glorious array of fresh fruits and vegetables.

Teeth that last must begin in prenatal life. Good structures require good foundations built solidly from the ample storehouses of protein, vitamins, and minerals. Positive nutrition for a lifetime, daily hygiene with proper brushing and flossing, and professional dental supervision will produce teeth that last.

Chapter 9

REDUCING HEALTH RISKS

Mortality studies clearly point to the degenerative diseases as the leading causes of death. Since most of these diseases cannot be cured, prevention seems to be the name of the game. This chapter will address some major health risks and problems, and will offer suggestions on how you can reduce the risks for these health problems.

Cancer

Recently the National Academy of Sciences' committee on diet, nutrition, and cancer evaluated a half century's collection of studies and literature on diet and cancer. The committee concluded: "The differences in rates at which various cancers occur in different human populations are often correlated with differences in diet. The likelihood that some of these correlations reflect causality is strengthened by laboratory evidence that similar dietary patterns and components of food also affect the incidence of certain cancers in animals."—*Diet, Nutrition, and Cancer* (Bethesda, Md.: National Cancer Institute).

The committee was unwilling to estimate how much diet actually contributes to overall cancer risks, nevertheless the members felt there was sufficient evidence to formulate these *interim* dietary guidelines:

1. Reduce intake of both saturated and unsaturated fats, from approximately 40 percent to approximately 30 percent total calories.

2. Include fruits, vegetables, and whole-grain cereal products in the daily diet, especially citrus fruits, dark-green and deep-yellow vegetables, and carotene-rich and brassica vegetables. Avoid high doses of dietary supplements. (Note: Brassica vegetables include turnips, kale, mustard greens, rutabaga, cauliflower, Brussels sprouts, and cabbage.)

3. Minimize consumption of cured, pickled, and smoked foods.

4. Use alcohol only in moderation. (Seventh-day Adventists

recommend total abstinence from alcohol.)

The committee found the strongest evidence for a connection between the amount of fat eaten and a higher risk of cancer, especially breast and colon cancer. Lacto-ovo-vegetarians who use low-fat milk and milk products and only moderate amounts of egg yolks and vegetable fats and oils may reduce their risk of various cancers.

The America Cancer Society's board of directors has launched a program to help reduce the risk of cancer. Its recommendations are summarized as follows:

1. Avoid obesity. Women 40 percent or more overweight had a 55 percent greater risk, and men a 33 percent greater risk, than normal.

2. Cut down on total fat intake. Not more than 30 percent of calories should come from fat.

3. Eat more high-fiber foods such as fruits, vegetables, and whole grains. Even though fiber itself may not protect against cancer, high-fiber foods are an excellent substitute for high-fat foods.

4. Include foods rich in vitamins A and C in the daily diet. (Capsule or tablet forms of these vitamins are not recommended.) Vitamin A foods—carotene-rich foods—are the dark-green and deep-yellow fruits and vegetables. Vitamin C foods are citrus fruits, tomatoes, green peppers, strawberries, cantaloupes, et cetera.

5. Include cruciferous (brassica) vegetables: cabbage, broccoli, Brussels sprouts, kohlrabi, and cauliflower. Some tests indicate that these foods may be highly effective in the prevention of chemically induced cancers.

6. Be moderate in consumption of alcoholic beverages. (Seventh-day Adventists recommend total abstinence from alcohol.)

7. Be moderate in consumption of salt-cured, smoked, and nitrite-cured foods.

Most of the suggestions outlined from these two institutions that have studied diet and cancer are natural outcomes of the lacto-ovo-vegetarian diet, a diet recommended by the Seventh-day Adventist Dietetic Association. Such a diet places emphasis on fruits, grains, nuts, seeds, and vegetables, and it eliminates all meat fats, caffeinated beverages, and alcohol.

Coronary Heart Disease

For twenty-five years the American Heart Association has continuously dialogued on the relationship between the American diet and coronary heart disease. And the dialogue is not finished yet, because new and complex information is emerging continually. In

1981 the American Heart Association published some dietary recommendations based on the concept that modification of risk factors should decrease the danger of heart disease. These risk factors are (1) elevated plasma cholesterol, (2) increased blood pressure, (3) smoking, (4) diabetes mellitus, and (5) marked obesity. To modify these risk factors, the American Heart Association makes these recommendations:

1. *Reduce intake of saturated fats.* The major sources of saturated fats are animal fat, meat, certain vegetable oils (palm oil, coconut oil, cocoa butter, and hydrogenated margarines and shortenings), butter fat (whole milk, cream, butter, ice cream, and cheese), and bakery goods. Lacto-ovo-vegetarians have already eliminated from their diet the two largest sources of saturated fat—animal fats and meat. In addition, if the butter fat is reduced by choosing low-fat milk and low-fat cheeses, a further significant reduction in saturated fat intake can be realized.

2. *Substitute unsaturated fats for saturated fats.* Although the free use of any fat is not recommended, it has been suggested that most of the separated fat eaten should be unsaturated. Unsaturated fats of choice are vegetable oils, except those mentioned in number 1.

3. *Increase the intake of carbohydrates.* If you reduce your fat intake by eating less of meat, full-fat dairy products, and ice cream, then you should eat more foods with complex carbohydrates—foods such as vegetables, beans, cereals, and fruits. These foods are a natural for the vegetarian.

4. *Substantially reduce dietary cholesterol.* The average meat-eating American consumes 450 to 500 milligrams of cholesterol per day. The American Heart Association recommends a reduction to 300 milligrams per day. The only source of dietary cholesterol is meat and animal fats. Lacto-ovo-vegetarians who eat only moderate amounts of egg yolks and use low-fat milk and milk products have significantly reduced their cholesterol intake.

5. *Adjust calorie intake to achieve and maintain desirable weight.* Diet-related risk factors are usually negatively affected by high-calorie diets and obesity. Vegetarians, on the average, have fewer problems with overweight than do their meat-eating peers.

It is not surprising, then, to discover that studies done on Seventh-day Adventists who were predominately lacto-ovo-vegetarians showed lower serum cholesterol levels and less coronary heart disease than control populations.

Caffeine

Many popular drinks (coffee, tea, cola, and certain other soft drinks) contain caffeine. Since caffeine is a true stimulant drug, it should be avoided. Caffeine increases the respiration rate, the heart rate, blood pressure, and the secretion of stress and other related hormones. Caffeine is habit-forming, and one's body will, to an extent, adapt to its effect. Continual use or overuse, however, can cause jittery feelings, nervousness, and gastric discomfort. An overdose can mimic the symptoms of an anxiety attack.

Caffeine is usually consumed for its "pick-up" effect. A far better replacement for a stimulant drug such as caffeine would be deep breathing, aerobic exercise for three to four minutes, or deep relaxation. Masking the symptoms of insufficient sleep by drinking coffee or cola all day does not promote health. Sooner or later the body's need for rest will have to be met if health is to be maintained.

Bone Mineral Loss

Osteoporosis is a "silent" disease that affects at least 25 percent of the female population and approximately one fourth of that number of males. Bones can lose calcium over a period of years, with no apparent symptoms. But when the pain resulting from the bone's becoming brittle is unrelenting, when the "dowager's hump" is visible to everyone, when inches of height are lost, and finally, when a hip breaks apparently without cause, *it is too late for dietary intervention.*

Again the lacto-ovo-vegetarian diet scores as a health asset. As stated in the mineral section of this text, vegetarians who have been studied lost much less bone mineral upon aging than people who were not vegetarians. Neither were they in the "fracture region" of mineral loss. Bones of these lifestyle vegetarians do not break easily.

Everyone loses bone mineral after about 35 years of age. To slow this deterioration process, people over 35 should adopt a diet that does not rob the bones of calcium, in order to maintain the blood neutrality that is essential to life.

A lifestyle that (1) includes a lacto-ovo-vegetarian diet begun early in life, (2) emphasizes calcium-containing foods, (3) follows a consistent exercise program, and (4) stresses drinking of water rather than alcohol, caffeinated, and carbonated beverages is another significant health risk reducer. Strong bone structure is the foundation of the body and the basis for vigor and lithe beauty.

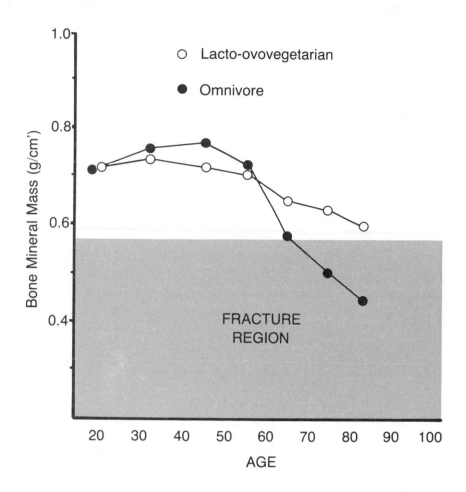

Mean bone mineral mass, calculated by decades of carefully matched pairs of lacto-ovo-vegetarians (open circles) and omnivores (filled circles). From Marsh *et al.*, with permission from *Journal of the American Dietetic Association*.

AN-7

Section III

Food Fundamentals
100/Food Puzzle Applied
115/Chemist in the Kitchen
120/Artist at Work

Chapter 10

FOOD PUZZLE APPLIED

Knowing the body's needs and the foods that will supply them is a great start on the road to good nutrition, but only what we actually eat will nourish us. Our goal must be to eat foods that (1) supply abundantly the nutrients needed, (2) please the eyes and the taste buds, and (3) stay within the budget. A big order? Yes, but you can simplify the task by choosing the necessary amounts from the Four Food Groups, by engaging in economical purchasing, and by carefully storing and preparing the food.

Fruit and Vegetable Group

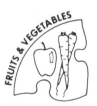

Colorful, mouth-watering fruits and vegetables add zest and delectability to daily meals. In this group lies the possibility of color to tempt the weary appetite, texture to please the dulled senses, aroma to stimulate gastric secretion, and an almost complete gamut of flavor. These foods add fiber to the diet. You can enjoy most fruits and vegetables as they are—delicious packages of vitamins, minerals, sugars, acids, and aromas.

Fruits and vegetables should appear fresh and in good condition when purchased, without any signs of spoilage. When you are choosing fruit such as citrus or pineapple, weight for size is important, because heavy ones hold more juice. Since fresh cabbage and head lettuce dehydrate with age, you can determine their quality by weight, also—the heavier, solid heads yield more servings. Soft spots, brown leaves, bruises, or deterioration around the stem or blossom end indicate poor quality. Seconds, as they are often called, can be purchased to advantage if the buyer has a specific purpose in mind to utilize them promptly, and if the price is reduced in proportion to the quality. Clean vegetables before refrigeration— preferably put them in plastic bags or in tight crispers as soon as possible. Curtailing purchasing and storage losses reduces price per serving.

During off-seasons, canned, frozen, and dried products often provide good buys and lend variety. Many ask, "Do canned and frozen fruits and vegetables have the same nutrients as fresh?" Modern processing procedures and jet-age transportation have helped make canned and frozen products very comparable in nutritive value with fresh products.

When purchasing, let the price per serving determine value. In comparing fresh, frozen, and canned fruits and vegetables, you will find, for example, that the waste in preparation of the fresh product and that the liquid on the canned product prohibit an ounce or pound comparison. As another example, two pounds of fresh peas in the pod equal one pound of frozen peas. The number of servings in a can is based on the drained contents. If a can of product and a package of frozen product yield the same number of servings, then compare prices. Dried fruits, seemingly high in price per pound, increase in volume with soaking and cooking, thus reducing cost per serving. When comparing prices, always ask, "How many servings will I get from this pound, can, or package?"

Both price and use should help determine the selection. The purpose intended will determine the quality or type of product to buy. For instance, fruit to be served whole and in its natural state should be more perfect than fruit cut up in salads or used in cooking. If inexpensive sliced peaches, small halves, and beautiful large halves in heavy syrup are available, the use makes a great difference when you are deciding which to buy. For arranged salads, you may want to choose the large halves, particularly if one half makes an attractive serving where otherwise two of the less expensive halves would be needed. Obviously, you would choose the slices for a cobbler in which you cut them up anyway. Generic foods with plain labels may prove quite satisfactory for some uses.

Fruits and vegetables at their best need little preparation. A good washing, perhaps scrubbing, removes germs, dust, and spray residues. Then they are ready to eat—delicious and attractive.

Cooking adds variety, and what a variety of possibilities exists, especially for vegetables! Pare and trim vegetables as little as possible, using a vegetable peeler to avoid excess waste and to conserve nutrients located directly under the skin. Young, tender vegetables may not need any peeling. All too often vegetables are boiled and buttered day after day, ignoring such possibilities as baking, roasting, frying, or combining various vegetables. Cooking not only increases variety in preparation, but hydrolyzes plant starch and makes it more digestible. Cooking also destroys microorganisms and stops enzyme action, slowing down spoilage.

If you do not utilize proper means of preparation, fruits and vegetables can lose their nutritive value. Skin provides a natural protective jacket that keeps nutrients in the food; hence, when you cook fruits and vegetables in the skins or in large pieces, they retain the most vitamins and minerals. Large pieces expose less surface area to the cooking water and air. However, if you can shorten the time of heating by exposing greater surface area, cutting fruits and vegetables into small pieces is justified.

Utilize the cooking water in soups, stews, or gravy; if stored for later use, seal the liquid, cool it immediately, and use it shortly. Never use soda to brighten green vegetables; it destroys B vitamins and oversoftens the vegetables. When cooking green vegetables, leave the lid off for the first three or four minutes of boiling, thus allowing the volatile acids to escape and preserving the green color. Add salt either first or last; however, it probably enhances flavor better when added first. If you desire margarine, add it at serving time.

About Nutrition

Generally use only a little water and a tight cover when cooking, but here again circumstances may alter the rule. Strongly flavored vegetables may be more acceptable if dropped into a large amount of boiling water and cooked quickly, with the cover off for at least the first few minutes to allow the strong odor to escape. You can cook vegetables high in water content—such as cabbage, onion, summer squash, and broccoli—in a Teflon or heavy skillet with a small amount of oil to prevent sticking. Stir them until they shrink, then turn down the heat, cover tightly, and let them steam in their natural juices.

A short cooking period maintains flavor, texture, and nutritive value. This applies to all vegetables. So-called waterless cooking may require a longer cooking time and result in more nutrient loss than when vegetables are cooked quickly in a moderate amount of water.

Bring water to a boil, add vegetables and salt, turn the heat down as soon as boiling starts, and continue cooking until the vegetables are tender but not mushy.

When you are cooking fruit, altering the time to add sugar produces different results. Fruit will maintain its shape if dropped into a boiling syrup and cooked gently. If you desire a sauce, cook the fruit first and then add sugar to the hot sauce, remembering that the fruit will taste sweeter when cold than while hot.

Although salads may consist of almost any food, they are most often composed of fruits and vegetables. A salad can serve as the appetizer, the main course, an accompaniment to the main course, or the dessert. It may be made from raw, frozen, or canned fruits or vegetables. It may be largely or partly protein food or even cereal. It may be cold or hot. It may be served in a large bowl and passed around, or it may be served as individual salads. In spite of all this variability, salads usually have three parts: the greens and/or garnish, the body, and the dressing.

The person who always uses head lettuce under the salad shows little imagination. Depending on the salad, leaf lettuce, deep-green spinach leaves, curly endive, watercress, or even celery leaves are attractive and tasty. The green base should be clean, crisp, dry, and fresh. It should never cover more than two thirds of the plate. A lettuce leaf split partway and folded over to make it into a cup is much more attractive than a flat, uninspired leaf.

Since the garnish provides a spot for creative individuality, surely other possibilities than maraschino cherries, parsley, and paprika will suggest themselves, though these are very useful. A bit of olive or pimiento, a sprig of watercress or mint, a wedge of apple or tomato, a slice of beet—these are some of the endless possibilities. Any attractive color contrast, with a compatible flavor, adds spark to the salad. But a little goes a long way!

The main part of the salad should usually have no more than three or four ingredients, placed casually or mixed. A salad arrangement that shows evidence of excessive handling indicates poor workmanship. Salads arranged to represent animals, faces, or other realistic things are not in good taste except for children or some special occasion. Refrigerate the complete salad or separate ingredients until the last minute if you plan to serve it cold.

Dressing and salad should complement each other. Why not add the dressing just before serving or pass it at the table? Macaroni, rice, some potato salads, and cooked vegetable salads may be marinated; that is, mix the dressing (usually French) with the salad ingredients far in advance of serving time—perhaps even the night before—so that flavors thoroughly blend. Refrigerate the marinating salad in a covered container.

In general there are three types of dressings: French, mayonnaise, and cooked. French dressing, the simplest type, is made of one-third lemon juice, two-thirds oil, or equal amounts of each, and seasonings such as a little sugar, salt, celery-and-onion salt, a dash of oregano, tomato puree, or whatever appeals. Put the ingredients into a small container with a tight cover, and shake. Some prepared French dressings have gums or powders added as emulsifiers to prevent separation of oil and acid. In addition to most of the above ingredients, mayonnaise contains egg yolk or whole egg as an emulsifier. Cooked dressings have a starch base. Dressing used to its best advantage brings out and adds to but does not drown the flavor of the salad.

Use the fruit and vegetable puzzle piece to splash color and variety onto the menu by following proper purchasing and preparation techniques.

Bread and Cereal Group

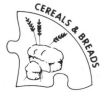

Grains form man's chief means of subsistence. Cereals and flours constitute as much as 80 percent of the diet in some countries. They play an important role in the low-cost diet because they store easily and because even in this country they cost the least. In the United States wheat is the most popular grain, being used for flours, cereals, and macaroni products. Use the common hard-wheat flours for breadmaking, and the all-purpose flour and soft-wheat flours for pastries and cake.

Barley, used for malt and interesting additions to soups and stews, is less popular. Small amounts of rye and buckwheat flours provide variety of flavor and texture in breadmaking. Rice may be the most versatile of the cereals, finding a natural spot in any meal of the day. Steamed rice as a breakfast cereal, rice pudding for dessert, and rice-and-vegetable casseroles reveal but a few of the possibilities.

You can use oats, usually considered a breakfast dish, in breads, dessert toppings, and as an extender in protein dishes. Corn, often considered a vegetable, is a grain used for cornmeal, grits, hominy, prepared cereal, cornstarch, and oil. Incorporating a variety of grains in the menu plan helps supply adequate vitamins and minerals. Many consider cooked cereals as breakfast foods, although their use need not be so limited.

Whole grains have three parts: the bran coats, germ, and endosperm. The bran coats contain fiber, B vitamins, and minerals. The germ furnishes the best quality protein of the grain, and the oil and vitamins. The endosperm is largely starch and protein. In the case of wheat and rye, this protein is gluten, an incomplete protein.

Refined grains contain only the endosperm. The bran and germ are removed in the milling process. This loss is serious because whole grains are one of the best sources of B vitamins. Most white flour and some other refined grain products have been "enriched" by adding thiamine, riboflavin, niacin, and iron. Whenever you use refined products, be sure they are enriched. The label will tell this. Even so, many of the B vitamins and other nutrients of the whole grains are not replaced. Whole grains are a much better buy nutritionally.

Fiber is important for a healthy digestive tract, to provide bulk. Fruits and vegetables also provide fiber, some of which may be digested. Most persons would not need a laxative if sufficient fiber was included in the foods they eat. Troubles such as hemorrhoids, diverticulosis, and perhaps even hiatus hernia and cancer of the colon might be prevented or alleviated.

Preparation of cereal foods often increases the price to consumers. In some cases they may cost too much, while some situations may justify the additional cost by saving time, storage space, and utilities. The homemaker should consider her time and facilities as expense whenever these are limited. Of the wide variety of convenience foods available in this group, sugar-coated breakfast cereals are the least desirable and most expensive. These cereals are highly refined, and while they may have some vitamins added, they do not compare favorably with whole-grain products.

Cooking raw cereal products increases the palatability, improves the appearance, and increases digestibility. Since the difference of degree and variety of preparation is so vast in the cereal group, rule-of-thumb instructions or cooking are not valid. Although the cooking directions on the package for hot cereals are the best guide, usually the less stirring, the better the results. To best cook regular rice, bring the water to boiling, add rice, and stir until each kernel of rice is separated, then turn the heat down, and cook the required time without removing the cover or stirring. Enriched products have had some nutrients restored after milling, so do not wash them before cooking.

Bread predominates in this group. Many consider it unnecessary to bake bread except for an occasional quick bread, yet how good it is to come home to the fragrant aroma of baking bread! Nothing so establishes the reputation of a good cook as a fine loaf of well-baked bread.

Breadmaking is no longer a tedious, uncertain process. Fresh yeasts, well-illustrated cookbooks, electric mixers, and easily controlled ovens make success possible even for the beginner. The yeast plant requires food, warmth, and moisture for growth. In breadmaking, stir or crumble the yeast into warm water containing a small amount of sugar. This supplies the three factors needed for growth. After the plant permeates the bread mixture, its enzymes convert some of the flour starch into the sugar the yeast needs for food, and it gives off carbon dioxide. The gluten of the flour stretches, holding in the gas formed and making the bread rise. When the bread is baking, the dough continues to rise for a few moments until it reaches a high-enough temperature to kill the yeast and coagulate the gluten protein.

Yeast, food for the yeast, and gluten are the essentials in breadmaking. Add sugar, aside from the starter for the yeast growth, in large or small amounts as desired. Brown sugar or molasses may be used for flavor instead of white sugar, but the amount used will not appreciably add to the nutritive value. Add salt to give bread a desirable flavor. Salt also controls yeast growth. However, salt-free bread can be made satisfactorily. Since only wheat flour and rye flour have sufficient gluten to make yeast bread, use other cereals and flours only as supplements. Use largely whole-wheat flour and other whole grains, but the beginner will find the dough easier to mix, and the finished product perhaps more acceptable to those unaccustomed to whole grains, if half of the flour is whole wheat and half is enriched white, gradually using more whole wheat and less white in later bakings. To boost the nutritive value, substitute up to one cup of dry or cooked oatmeal, cornmeal, or other cereal or flour per loaf. When using soy flour, substitute only one-fourth cup per loaf. The fat used to make the bread more tender may be oil, margarine, or solid shortening.

Following a formula for breadmaking allows the baker to use the foods on hand and gives a variety of delicious breads. The following formula will make one loaf:

    1 cake or pkg. yeast (enough for up to 4 loaves)

    1¼ cups water (fruit or vegetable or tomato juice may be substituted for a taste treat)

    1 to 2 Tbsp. sugar, white or brown, or molasses

    1 to 2 Tbsp. fat

    1 to 1½ tsp. salt

    3 to 3½ cups flour, at least 2 to 2½ cups of which is wheat flour

Any standard bread recipe explains the method of mixing. For a crisp crust as in French bread, brush the top of the bread with egg white diluted with one to two tablespoonfuls of water. Brush the bread once before baking and one after it has baked twenty minutes.

Oat Rolls

    1¼ cups boiling water

    2 Tbsp. oil

    2 Tbsp. brown sugar

    1 tsp. salt

    1 cup oatmeal

    1 pkg. dry yeast

    ¼ cup warm water

    2 cups whole-wheat flour

    2 cups white flour (enriched)

    1 egg

Pour boiling water over oil, sugar, salt, and oats, letting stand until lukewarm. Sprinkle yeast over the warm water and stir to dissolve. Add 2 cups flour and the egg to oat mixture. Mix and add yeast gradually. Add remaining flour. Knead 5 to 10 minutes. Let rise until double in bulk, about 1½ hours. Punch down, form rolls, and let rise again about ½ hour. Bake at 350° F. about 25 minutes.

Many people do not use products containing soda and baking powder, for generally such products (cakes, cookies, quick breads, et cetera) are less healthful because of the excess sugar and fat they contain in addition to the leavening product. For those who do choose to use baking soda and baking powder, here are a few principles to follow:

    1. Soda must be neutralized with an acid. Many recipes do not do this. Unneutralized soda becomes washing soda when heated and is very irritating to the stomach. It also destroys B vitamins. One-half teaspoon of soda will be neutralized with one of the following:

        a. One cup fully soured milk or buttermilk

        b. One tablespoon lemon juice

     c. Three-fourths cup dark molasses

     d. One-fourth teaspoon cream of tartar

  2. Baking powder is soda plus an acid and cornstarch. It contains sufficient acid to neutralize the soda.

     a. One teaspoon baking powder is sufficient to leaven one cup sifted flour.

     b. If the recipe calls for more soda than can be neutralized as suggested above, one teaspoon baking powder may be substituted for each one-half teaspoon soda not neutralized by acid ingredients.

     c. Baking powder must be kept dry and not exposed to air longer than necessary. Close the can immediately after measuring the amount needed.

     d. Buy in small quantity. Stir before measuring. Do not use if it becomes lumpy.

The jigsaw piece depicting cereals and breads fits neatly into the food puzzle and offers a diverse supply of tastes and textures while contributing necessary nutrients to the daily meal plan.

Protein Group

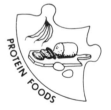

All foods in the Four Food Groups contain some protein, but the amount of protein in one serving determines those to include in this group. The protein group includes meat, yellow cheese, cottage cheese, wheat gluten, nuts, eggs, and legumes—dried peas, beans, garbanzos (chick-peas), and peanuts.

Each food in the group contains specific proteins, some complete and some incomplete, which require supplementation. Wheat gluten and legumes (with the possible exception of soybeans) furnish incomplete proteins. They do not individually furnish all the essential amino acids necessary to make a complete protein that the body requires for building and repair. However, these vegetable proteins in combination can supplement one another. They are well supplemented when used with even small amounts of egg or dairy

ABOUT NUTRITION

products, which do contain complete proteins. Many of the commercial canned and frozen protein foods available are formulated so that ingredients supplement one another. (See section in chapter 3 on the supplementation of proteins.)

Meat is a protein so commonly used that nutritionists often call the whole protein group "the meat group," but this does not bestow upon it top priority. In some countries, meat comprises only a small portion of the diet. Meat costs run high in terms of money and land required to produce it, and replacing meat with vegetable proteins may become necessary as populations explode and farmlands decrease. Meat analogs, as vegetable proteins are often called—produced from spun soy protein, wheat protein (called gluten), or from food combinations—make satisfactory entrées, supplying a good portion of the day's protein needs.

You can purchase legumes—which provide an inexpensive source of protein—raw, dried, or ready to eat. Make the raw and dried ones edible by cooking them to soften the cellulose and facilitate the utilization of their protein. Make wheat gluten from pure-gluten flour or high-gluten flour, or purchase gluten ready to eat in a vast variety of sizes, shapes, and flavors. Meat analogs cost less per edible pound than meat. They have little fat and no bone waste and do not shrink. These foods are tasty, nutritious, easy to prepare, and can replace meat in many recipes.

Eggs should be clean, without crack, and fresh or stored under quality conditions. Shell color or shape, unless extreme, does not affect the quality. Medium-sized eggs usually provide the best buy for household use.

A few general characteristics apply to this group as a whole. All proteins coagulate, or set, when heated. Previous to heating they can be stretched. They form foams and can be denatured; that is, heating or additions of sugar or salt can change their characteristics. Too rapid heating toughens them.

Effective preparation of proteins involves consideration of the previously mentioned characteristics. Wash dried legumes—beans, peas, and lentils—and soak them so that they swell and absorb water. If you cannot soak them overnight, heat them to the boiling point in about three cups of water to one cup of legumes, remove from the heat, and soak for one hour before cooking. Boil or pressure-cook soaked legumes. Soybeans in particular require long cooking if pressure is not used.

Gluten, the main protein substance found in wheat, may be extracted and used to make entrées with meatlike texture and flavor.

To make gluten, knead bread flour and water to a smooth dough, cover with water, and allow to set a half hour or more. Then wash the starch out, kneading under water; change the water several times. (No washing is required when 100 percent gluten flour is used. Follow directions on package.) A very elastic mass—the gluten—remains. Drop chunks or slices of gluten into boiling flavored broth; this causes them to swell promptly and then coagulate. Simmer the gluten slowly from this point for an hour to absorb both broth and flavor and to cook the protein without toughening it. If you desire a more tender product, leave in a small quantity of starch during the washing process, to separate the gluten strands.

Since legume protein adequately supplements wheat protein, adding soy flour or mashed legumes to a gluten loaf is a good procedure. Small amounts of milk or eggs supplement cereal and legume protein. Nuts and brewer's yeast also supplement to some extent the protein of legumes. However, since nuts are very high in fat, use them only in small quantities. A guideline given in 1901 still applies to their use today: "One-tenth to one-sixth part of nuts would be sufficient, varied according to combinations."—Ellen G. White, *Counsels on Diet and Foods,* p. 365.

One egg provides six grams of complete protein. But remember that egg yolks are high in cholesterol and should be limited to not more than three a person each week. Egg whites may be used more generously if you desire. When preparing eggs, always gently but thoroughly cook them. Because eggs provide an excellent growth medium for bacteria, thick meringues, egg white beaten into cooked puddings, or raw eggs used in any fashion are not safe. Cook them at least five minutes. The Food and Drug Administration now requires pasteurization of all eggs and egg products sold outside the shell. Always cook eggs gently by simmering, not boiling. The rapid boiling of eggs is neither desirable nor necessary. In fact, the hard boiling of any food except when evaporating liquid is not a good cooking practice.

Dairy products such as ice cream and cheese may be included in the protein group if eaten in addition to the amount recommended in the milk group. Cottage cheese greatly adds variety, for it fits in so many places—salads, main dishes, even desserts. Vegetarian cookbooks contain recipes for a wide variety of tasty, nutritious protein foods.

This important puzzle piece appears complicated because of its many-faceted components, but to summarize, always cook proteins gently. Soaking benefits legume and gluten proteins. Nuts supply a good protein, but use them sparingly because of high-fat content. Combining proteins offers a desirable way to provide all essential amino acids.

Milk Group

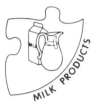

Milk is a food, and as such, definitely use it with the meal. Containing 13 percent solids, milk has less water than cabbage, berries, summer squash, and greens.

Milk can be purchased in many forms:

1. Homogenized whole milk. This contains 3 to 4 percent butterfat and is fortified with vitamins A and D.

2. Two percent milk—actually, 2 percent fat milk. A part of the butterfat has been removed. Otherwise all the nutrients of whole milk are retained.

3. Fluid skim milk. In skim milk practically all the fat has been removed; nonfat dry milk powder may be added. All the other nutrients are retained.

4. Nonfat dry milk powder. It consists of milk from which the fat and the water have been removed. This dried powder is most often sold in an "instant" form, which mixes with water readily. In some places a form that requires a blender or beater for mixing may be purchased. This is less expensive and is labeled "noninstant." While one and one-third cups of the instant powder are required for one quart of milk, only one cup of the noninstant is needed per quart. Nonfat dry milk may be used in baking and cooking without reconstituting. It should be added with the other dry ingredients, and water substituted in the recipe for the liquid milk specified. Reconstituted nonfat dry milk may be chilled for a very acceptable beverage. The only nutritional difference is the absence of cream—the butterfat.

5. Evaporated milk. This is milk from which slightly more than half the water has been evaporated. One thirteen-ounce can is equal to one quart of whole milk in nutrients. The milk is sterilized in the

can, and some persons who cannot tolerate other milk can use this. Lactose, the sugar in milk, carmelizes when heated. This fact, coupled with carbon dioxide loss during heating, gives evaporated milk its distinctive flavor. Evaporated milk is excellent for cooking because it does not curdle as easily as fresh milk. If thoroughly chilled, it may be whipped to produce a topping or to take the place of whipped cream in salads and desserts. It supplies much less fat and more protein than does rich cream and may be used instead of cream.

6. Raw milk. It is not generally safe for human use. All milk should be pasteurized.

7. Sweetened condensed milk. The water has been evaporated as in evaporated milk, and a large amount of sugar has been added.

Commercial fortified soy beverages now available are particularly valuable for those allergic to milk. The same milk cookery principles apply when you are cooking with the soy product, since it is a protein food.

In choosing milk, consider cost and nutritive values. To analyze price, compare price and nutritive value of the equivalent of a quart of fresh milk.

Milk, as a protein food, requires a special cooking technique. Cook it gently in a double boiler or in a heavy kettle over low heat. Stir it frequently to prevent it from sticking, scorching, and forming skin. The skin forming on the top and the part sticking to the bottom and sides of the pan are calcium caseinate, calcium, and protein. The foam that forms when you reconstitute dry milk contains much protein. Allow it to settle instead of discarding it.

Yogurt

    3 cups warm water (approximately 85° F.)
1½ cups nonfat dry milk
    ¼ cup plain yogurt

Mix the ingredients thoroughly. Pour into containers (4 to 5 oz.), and cover tightly. Process in yogurt maker, or set jars in warm water in an electric frying pan set at 150° F. Let stand 5 or 6 hours. Remove containers and refrigerate.

Use in salad dressings, in place of sour cream in recipes, or eat with fruit. Delicious with a tablespoon of frozen orange juice concentrate.

Frozen Lemon Dessert

    1 can (13 oz.) evaporated milk
    ⅓ cup lemon juice
    ⅓ to ½ cup sugar (to taste)

Graham cracker crumbs

Chill the milk in the freezer until ice crystals form around the edge. Whip until peaks form when the beaters are lifted. Add lemon juice and sugar. Mix and spoon over graham cracker crumbs. Sprinkle top with a few cracker crumbs. Return to freezer for several hours. Slice to serve.

Having examined the last piece of the puzzle, you may discover a favorite food or combination of foods missing. The Four Food Groups pattern does not have a dessert group, for desserts are not essential for growth or maintenance of good health. Persons accustomed to finishing a meal with something sweet may find that a piece of fruit will satisfy this desire. Include milk desserts in the milk group if you consider the actual amount of milk to be significant. Avoid the dessert that furnishes only calories when too many have already been consumed, or the dessert that crowds out the day's Four Food Group requirements. Pies and cakes do have a place as a treat now and then, but consider them only as treats. The addition of honey, whole-wheat or soy flour, dates, or nuts will *not* turn a rich sweet dessert into a health food that you may eat freely.

Beverages play an important role in the diet. Fruit and vegetable juices are good, though the whole fruit or vegetable has the advantage of the whole package rather than just the juice. Use unsweetened fruit juices more than the highly sweetened and artificially flavored fruit drinks. Many beverages (such as Hi-C or Tang) contain only a small amount of fruit juice or none at all. Read labels. Remember that ingredients are listed in order of amounts in the product. Chocolate and cocoa also have some nutritive value and are not as habit-forming as tea and coffee. Carob is sometimes used instead of cocoa. However, its very high sugar content scarcely makes it more desirable from a health standpoint. If it is used, the sugar in the recipe should be reduced. One problem with using large quantities of chocolate is that it contains much more fat than cocoa, which has had a portion of the cocoa butter removed. When chocolate, cocoa, or carob are used as beverages, consider them in the dessert class. Because of the high sugar content, also limit carbonated soft drinks in the well-managed diet. Hot cereal beverages and some herb teas, free of caffeine, are enjoyable during cool weather or served at social occasions. Of the many beverages available, the essential Four Food Groups include only milk and fruit and vegetable juices. Choose these beverages for nutritional value. They require little preparation and contribute pleasantly and rewardingly to good nutrition.

AN-8

Of all drinks, water quenches thirst best. In drinking, as in eating, develop good habits. Water, although not listed in the Four Food Groups, is essential to positive health, in quantities of at least six cups a day.

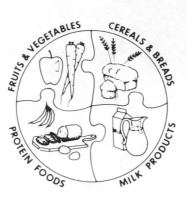

The food puzzle correctly put together presents a picture of complete nutrition for the body's needs. Time spent in careful purchasing allows everyone the correct amounts from the Four Food Groups puzzle, on even a limited food budget. Proper storage prevents loss of quality and nutritive value. Skillful preparation of food assures that each needed nutrient is consumed every day so that the nutrition puzzle does not fail of completion.

Chapter 11

CHEMIST IN THE KITCHEN

Similar to the way the matrix makes the preschool puzzle workable is the work of the chemist in the kitchen, who sets the foundation for acceptance or rejection of the food puzzle pieces. The complex foods, which provide nutrition for the body, have both chemical and physical properties that react variously during preparation and cooking processes. These reactions produce diverse results as cooking progresses.

As the laboratory chemist accurately measures and combines the chemicals for a desired reaction, so the chemist in the kitchen must follow directions exactly to achieve uniformly good results.

A standard cookbook gives recipes in a form easily read and followed. It lists the ingredients in order of use, with precise instructions, and gives size of servings and yield per recipe. The cookbook's size and shape should warrant easy storage. Pages that open flat and stay open for quick reference have their advantage. The recipes should use ingredients and utensils found in the average kitchen. Of what value is a recipe, no matter how delicious, that requires items one does not have on hand or expensive equipment one cannot afford? The gourmet cook may choose additional books or a collection of exotic recipes.

A good index saves much time, and the cookbook should include a glossary of terms used in food preparation. The experienced meal manager will find a table of weights and measures helpful when cooking or when preparing a shopping list.

A table of equivalents helps one determine how much raw food yields a specific measured amount. An example:

Bread crumbs   3 to 4 slices dry bread = 1 cup dry crumbs
                    1 slice fresh bread = ¾ cup soft crumbs

A table of substitutions can help when you are preparing a recipe and do not have a necessary ingredient. An example:

Milk   1 cup whole milk =   1 cup reconstituted nonfat dry milk plus 2 teaspoons butter, margarine, or oil

If you want to experiment with vegetable protein, use the section on meat cookery as a guide, since vegetable protein foods can substitute for meat in many popular recipes, such as vegetarian lasagna and stroganoff. Additional desirable features in a cookbook include menu suggestions, guides to preparation, and illustrations. Pictures provide inspiration and ideas for serving. A good cookbook with good recipes is the laboratory manual for the kitchen chemist.

Careless *measuring* is probably the most common reason for recipe failure. Money spent for standard measuring equipment is wisely invested. Measuring spoons, graduated dry measuring cups (¼, ⅓, ½, 1 cup), a good metal spatula, and a glass or plastic cup with a rim above the one-cup line for liquid measure are recommended. An experienced cook with his personal recipes may obtain good results using nonstandardized methods of measuring, but even then the product might not turn out the same each time.

For accuracy, level measuring spoons and dry measuring cups with a spatula. Table-service spoons and teacups do not measure accurately. Spoon flour lightly into a cup without headspace and level off. Sifting before measuring gives greater accuracy and is recommended when the recipe designates sifted flour. The unsifted cup of flour contains about two tablespoons more flour than the sifted. This extra flour can cause dryness, peaking, and cracking in baked products.

Liquid-measuring cups need headspace above the one-cup mark to avoid spilling. For accuracy, read the amount in the cup at eye level with the cup on the counter. In recipes including one or more eggs, use medium-sized eggs. When you divide in half a recipe calling for one egg, beat the egg thoroughly and use half the total volume.

Measure solid fat by packing it into a dry measuring cup, leaving no air space, or measure it by water displacement. If, for instance, you need one-half cup of fat, fill a liquid measuring cup with cold water to the one-half-cup mark. Add shortening and push below the water until the water reaches the one-cup mark. Then pour off the water if not needed in the recipe. The shortening will slip out easily and completely.

Many factors other than the ingredients in the recipe also affect the finished product. *Manipulation, or handling,* may cause wide variation. Consider the beating of egg white, for example. First, a foam of large bubbles forms. Gradually the foam becomes finer and begins to stiffen. When the beater is lifted and a soft peak forms that turns over slightly, the greatest volume is reached. With continued beating, the peaks become stiff and dry, and the volume somewhat decreases. Decided overbeating produces little volume with white specks of congealed egg white. A recipe requiring one stage of beating will not produce an ideal product with another stage.

Stirring and kneading a flour mixture develop the gluten—desirable in breadmaking but undesirable in muffins and pastry. Overstirring causes tunnels in muffins and results in tough pastry. Insufficient kneading of dough produces poor quality bread. Adequate creaming of sugar and fat is necessary for acceptable butter cakes and cookies.

The *type and size of pan* are important. You cannot obtain a standard product when using an oversize or undersize pan. Using an oversize pan for whipping egg whites or cream results in poor volume. For range-top cooking, flat-bottom pans that completely cover the heating element conduct the heat best. A pan that is too small for the burner wastes energy.

Glass, iron, or dark tin causes products to bake more quickly and burn more easily than a shiny tin or aluminum pan. A baking sheet with sides will cause cookies on the outer edge to burn before the ones in the center are baked. If you use such a pan, turn it over and use the bottom for baking. Bake most drop cookies on an ungreased cookie sheet and remove them from the sheet a few minutes after you take them from the oven. Teflon-coated bake pans require no greasing and clean very easily.

Some factors not listed as ingredients affect recipe results. Consider *air,* for example. It conducts heat slowly, as in baking; it causes browning of fruits and vegetables. Covering to shut out the air or dipping in acid such as lemon or pineapple juice somewhat prevents browning. Oxygen in the air destroys vitamin C, whereas the acid and/or covering helps retain it. Air also doubles as a leavening agent—the only one in angel food cake. The egg whites hold the air bubbles, which expand when heated. First the egg white stretches and then coagulates. Creaming the sugar and shortening also entraps some air. The grains of sugar are porous, and the shortening surrounding them shuts in the air. This helps make some baked products light.

Water conducts heat faster than air and prevents burning. It can help to prevent the darkening of peeled vegetables by shutting out the air. It often becomes an ingredient without adding flavor. Too much water, of course, reduces flavor and nutrients. Water softens, dissolves, and aids in mixing. Pure water boils at a constant temperature. Adding dissolvable substances changes the boiling point. Rapid boiling does not shorten cooking time; it only breaks up food, evaporates water, and often causes the food to burn. Once the water boils, turn down the heat to the temperature that will continue the cooking gently. One exception to this is in making jelly or candy, where rapid boiling brings about the desired result. Here it increases the concentration of dissolved substances as it boils the water away.

Another factor is *temperature*. Ingredients blend best but spoil quickly at room temperature. Heat destroys bacteria; freezing inactivates them; refrigerator temperatures slow down bacterial growth. Heat transfers more quickly through oil or shortening in frying than through water in boiling or air in baking.

Less fat is absorbed in deep-fat frying than in panfrying if the fat is in good condition and is held at the right temperature (a thermometer is essential for deep-fat frying if the fryer is not automatic), and if pieces are fairly large. Fat in good condition has never smoked and is clear and odorless. Too-high temperatures cause smoking and chemical breakdown. Too-low temperatures allow the food to absorb too much fat and become soggy. Strain the fat after each use, as crumbs and pieces cause it to break down, developing harmful substances and causing greater absorption. Automatic electric frying pans take the guesswork out of panfrying in a small amount of fat. Teflon-coated pans require no fat to prevent sticking.

When heat is applied to food, (1) water evaporates, causing loss of weight and greater concentration of the food; (2) protein coagulates, or sets; (3) starch swells as it absorbs water; (4) fat melts; (5) cellulose softens; (6) colors and flavors change, a browning reaction may occur, and sugars caramelize; (7) some vitamins are lost; and (8) many complex chemical and physical interactions take place other than the more simple ones commonly recognized.

Altitude also affects cooking processes. At a high altitude the boiling temperature lowers, and the pressure cookers become very important to reach a high-enough temperature to get foods done. Always adjust the pressure pan for altitude. You may have to alter recipes to include more strengthening ingredients, such as flour and eggs, and less weakening ingredients, such as baking powder, sugar, and fat. Depending on the altitude, increase liquid in baked products by one to four tablespoons per cup of liquid, owing to more rapid evaporation in higher altitudes. Biscuits and muffins require less adjustment than cakes with a more delicate structure. Obtain recipes for baking at high altitudes and information regarding cooking from the agriculture stations of many high-altitude States. Cake mixes often include suggestions for baking at high altitudes.

Acids and alkalies may cause decided color and texture changes. Sometimes they are present in foods and water, or they may be added. Examples of acids in food are ascorbic acid in lemon juice, acetic acid in vinegar, and citric acid in citrus fruit. Acids toughen fibers, turn greens brown, whiten whites, and brighten reds. If you flavor a vegetable with lemon juice, add it after cooking to prevent toughening.

Alkalies cause fibers to weaken and greens to remain bright, but affect other colors unfavorably—reds turn blue or green, and whites turn yellow. Alkalies destroy vitamin C and the B vitamins, whereas acids protect them. The most common alkali used in cooking is baking soda. The use of soda and baking powder in baked products is discussed in chapter 10. Never add soda to vegetables because it destroys vitamins.

Through everyday experiments, the kitchen chemist observes the many reactions resulting from chemical and physical properties of the foods in the Four Food Groups. Some reactions please; others are disastrous. Some of the food-puzzle pieces are delicate, others hardy. Accurate kitchen equipment and an increasing knowledge of food preparation principles assure the chemist of desired results.

Chapter 12

ARTIST AT WORK

In the artist's mind, a picture matures, combining color, balance, and form into a lovely creation. The food artist, understanding family needs for good nutrition and the principles of food preparation, sets to work. Colors, shapes, flavors, and textures of food furnish components for the masterpiece. The basic sketch for pleasing meals evolves from a well-thought-out and visualized menu, the table setting, and the surroundings; even the people partaking of the meal form the background.

Mealtimes—When and Where?

To successfully plan menus, first of all determine time and place for the meals, for circumstances dictate mealtimes. Where schedules remain flexible, two meals a day constitute an excellent plan for relatively inactive adults. When work or school schedules dictate three meals a day, it is ideal to serve the main meal at midday, with a light meal in the evening. When the family is not together at noon, make the evening meal substantial enough to provide the remaining food needs of the day. A well-designed meal schedule discourages the current trend of frequent snacks.

Plan a hearty first meal every day. Skipping breakfast or eating skimpy breakfasts robs many fine productive hours from the morning. Midmorning letdown, accompanied by the temptation to fortify oneself with the empty calories of sweet rolls or doughnuts, usually occurs about ten o'clock. Breakfastless individuals work below capacity until the noon meal takes effect in midafternoon. This trend has become so apparent and serious that some communities give children breakfast or at least orange juice and/or milk on arrival at school. Successful home artists strive to make breakfast so appealing that no one will want to miss it.

If the main meal must be at night, serve it as early as possible. Children usually arrive home from school hungry. A large meal at this time or soon after could solve the snack problem and the late evening meal problem.

In many places school lunch programs do a splendid job of providing adequate noonday meals. Carried lunches can definitely contribute to the daily nutritional needs if you use a variety of menus such as "A Month's Suggestions for Pack-It Lunches" on page 122 advocates. Drab, monotonous lunches disappear when the thoughtful artist takes over.

Home remains the most popular place to eat. What better memories of home can one carry with him than visions of the family gathering around the dining table and chattering about the day's activities? Must you always serve home meals in the kitchen or the dining room? No. More and more families like to eat on the patio, in the living room, or wherever they enjoy being together. Some meals you will eat away from home, at school, at work, or when traveling. Some you will eat out just for fun.

Four Food Groups in Menus

"What shall we have for supper?" leads to frustration if you leave the answer until a few minutes before mealtime. Planning ahead requires a few extra minutes, but it eventually saves both time and money. It saves time in shopping, preparation, and avoiding that wondering-what-to-prepare period. Institutions successfully use cycle menus; why not adapt such for home use? Repeat a three- or four-week cycle of menus over and over with changes for seasons, holidays, or other special occasions. Perhaps it seems that reusing the same menu means traveling in a rut, but the monotonous rut dredges even deeper with no planning. Getting the meal plan on paper enables the homemaker to see the job as a whole, and avoid dreary repetitions day after day without a menu. A cycle menu should never limit the homemaker, but provide security, while allowing freedom and flexibility.

The menu planner needs a place to work, preferably in the kitchen. Provide the needed tools—a file of favorite recipes, cookbooks, pictures, new recipes to try, a sharp pencil, and eraser. To keep your file useful, weed out the recipes never used. Basic cookbooks contain lists of salads, main dishes, and desserts, ways to prepare vegetables, and other menu suggestions.

Good nutrition requires top priority in menu planning. Including a wide variety from the Four Food Groups every day is a good means of accomplishing this. The four servings of fruits and vegetables will probably divide up into vegetables at the main meal and fruit at breakfast and supper or lunch. Oranges, grapefruit, or their juices

A Month's Suggestions for Pack-It Lunches

Something Hearty	Something Crisp	Something Toothsome	Something Drinkable	Something to Surprise (optional)
FIRST WEEK				
Mon. Peanut butter sandwich	Carrot strips	Applesauce	Potato soup (cream)	Dried fruit
Tues. Nutmeat-spread sandwich	Cucumber sticks	Orange, quartered	Milk	Date bar
Wed. Egg sandwich	Celery sticks	Apple, quartered	Milk	Fruit candy
Thurs. Vegesteak sandwich	Assorted relishes	Fruit salad	Tomato juice	Oatmeal cookie
Fri. Tomato-and-lettuce sandwich	Olives	Half banana	Milk	Bag of salted peanuts
SECOND WEEK				
Mon. Soy cheese sandwich	Cucumber sticks	Apple, quartered	Tomato soup (cream)	Fruit whip
Tues. Egg sandwich	Lettuce wedge	Jelled fruit salad	Milk	Peanut butter cookie
Wed. Bean sandwich	Olives	Apricots (fresh or canned)	Fruit juice	Cupcake
Thurs. Tomato-and-lettuce sandwich	Stuffed celery	Half banana	Milk	Mixed nuts
Fri. Peanut butter sandwich	Carrot sticks	Berries (fresh or frozen)	Milk	Pudding
THIRD WEEK				
Mon. Vegetable wiener on bun	Nuts	Cherries (fresh or canned)	Milk	Dried fruit
Tues. Tomato-and-lettuce sandwich	Olives	Orange, quartered	Milk	Stuffed prunes
Wed. Cottage cheese	Crackers	Tomato, quartered	Vegetable soup	Molasses cookie
Thurs. Egg sandwich	Celery curls	Ripe pear	Milk	Fruit whip
Fri. Savory garbanzo sandwich	Carrot sticks	Pineapple chunks	Milk	Dates
FOURTH WEEK				
Mon. Hard-boiled egg (deviled)	Assorted relishes	Potato salad, crackers	Milk	Dried fruit
Tues. Vegeburger on bun	Carrot strips	Peaches (fresh or canned)	Milk	Pudding
Wed. Tomato-and-lettuce sandwich	Stuffed celery	Melon, peeled and sliced	Milk	Coconut cookie
Thurs. Peanut butter sandwich	Olives	Grapes	Fruit juice	Rice pudding
Fri. Egg sandwich	Lettuce wedge	Half banana	Tomato soup (cream)	Dried fruit

Reprinted from L. Sonnenberg, ed., *Everyday Nutrition for Your Family*, p. 42.

served at breakfast will provide the daily serving of high vitamin C food. Tomatoes, strawberries, cantaloupe, raw or lightly cooked cabbage, broccoli, or even new potatoes cooked in the jacket may take the place of citrus fruit on occasion. Greens, broccoli, asparagus, carrots, sweet potatoes, squash, or pumpkin can serve as the deep-green or dark-yellow vegetable. One every other day from this group efficiently supplies vitamin A. Consider one-half cup of a cooked fruit or vegetable an adult serving.

The four servings of cereal and bread may include a cereal at breakfast and one or more slices of toast. This group includes macaroni, spaghetti, noodles, and rice, but they should not frequently replace potatoes, as potatoes supply needed minerals. A cereal dish is a good idea for supper or lunch to ensure the four servings required.

Each meal needs a good source of protein. Cereals, bread, and milk throughout the day, with two servings of foods high in protein—one at dinner, the other at breakfast or supper—will meet this need. Do not exempt cottage cheese, vegetable-protein food, legumes, or nuts from breakfast. Custom alone dictates that an egg constitutes the only protein food suitable for breakfast. If you expect entrées to supply the protein needs of the meal, make certain they contain sufficient amounts of good-quality protein. If a serving will not provide two or three ounces of a protein food, a salad made from cottage cheese, or legumes such as peas or lima beans, can supplement the entrée. Do not consider a dish made largely of macaroni or bread crumbs and seasoning a protein food.

The required amount of milk includes milk used in cooking. One-half cup of ice cream or milk pudding supplies a half serving of milk. Milk gravies, soups, and creamed vegetables add their share. One-half cup of undiluted evaporated milk equals one cup of whole milk.

Good meal planning begins with the day's main meal. First of all, select the main dish or protein dish, then the vegetables, salad, and dessert if you plan to serve one. Only three or four dishes a meal are needed, even when inviting company to dinner—a protein dish; a starchy dish, such as potatoes, corn, macaroni, spaghetti, noodles, or rice; a cooked vegetable; and a salad or raw vegetable sticks. Casserole dishes, stews, or even salads including several vegetables and a good quantity of protein may furnish all the nutrients for a fine one-dish meal, with something raw and crisp as a side dish. Too much variety tempts one to overeat.

The remaining meal or meals should include selections to round out the Four Food Groups and ensure good nutrition for the day.

A Pattern for Meal Planning

	Light	Hearty
Breakfast	Fruit Cereal and milk or Protein (egg or other) Bread and butter	Fruits (2) Cereal and cream Protein (egg or other) Bread and butter or waffles, pancakes, doughnuts, etc. Milk
Dinner	Protein dish Starchy vegetable or other Cooked vegetable (green or yellow) Salad or raw vegetable Milk or other beverage	Protein dish Starchy vegetable (or other starchy food, as macaroni) Two cooked vegetables (one green or yellow) Salad Bread and butter Milk or other beverage Dessert
Lunch or Supper	Soup, salad, or cereal Sandwich, bread and butter, or crackers Fruit Milk	Soup and crackers Salad Sandwich or bread and butter Fruit Milk

---

Adapted from Bogert, Briggs, and Calloway, *Nutrition and Physical Fitness*, 8th ed., pp. 494-496.

Breakfast need not follow a set pattern, but the average breakfast includes a fruit, cereal or egg, bread or toast, and milk. Supper or lunch may consist of a main dish—such as a casserole, soup, a hearty sandwich cold or hot, or cereal—and suitable fruit, bread, and beverage accompaniments. Page 124 gives some menu patterns for light and hearty meals.

In addition to furnishing adequate nutrition, meals should satisfy the appetite and please the diners. Adequate utilization of the simple food puzzle—this includes providing protein at every meal and the inclusion of some fats such as butter, margarine, or oil satisfy the body's needs and appetite. Fat and protein provide satiety because they digest more slowly and take more time to metabolize than do starches and sugars.

Pleasing the diner merits consideration. Family likes and dislikes will and should influence the menus. Teaching children to like a wide variety of food comprises an important part of fitting them for life, for good nutrition, and for social acceptability. A hostess and mother appreciates the guest and family who truly enjoy the food she prepares. However, allow every person to dislike a food or two. In writing menus do not entirely omit disliked foods, but serve them occasionally so that the family may learn to enjoy them. Buying large quantities of disliked foods wastes storage space and money, whereas small portions served in a variety of ways with well-liked foods give an unknown or disliked food its best chance for acceptance.

Aesthetic appeal dictates that each meal should contain variety in flavor, form, texture, and color. Foods of only one color or shape do not make an attractive meal. Serving corn, peas, and beans at the same meal or choosing four dishes each with a sauce or gravy does not appeal. Complement soft foods such as mashed potatoes, loaves, and soft vegetables with crispy and crunchy foods. Cooked vegetables can add texture if not overcooked. Use only one strong-flavored vegetable at a meal.

If you plan at least a week's menus at one time on a large sheet of paper, you will more easily visualize the meals and detect repetition of shape, color, and flavor. Avoid repeating a food on the same day unless in a very different form. Page 126, "Common Errors in Meal Planning and How to Correct Them," illustrates these suggestions.

Freezers provide service in taking care of leftovers and holding them at acceptable quality until they again become new to the eyes of the family. "Planned overs" remunerate menu makers. For example, leftover lentil roast from today becomes sliced sandwich filling later in the menu cycle. Or you may utilize the remaining burger from one

Common Errors in Meal Planning and How to Correct Them

Poor	Better
1. TOO MANY STARCHES	
Noodles with soya chicken	Noodles with soya chicken
Mashed potatoes	Spinach
Corn	Sliced tomatoes
Bean salad	Crisp cookies
Rice pudding	
2. TOO MUCH PROTEIN	
Macaroni and cheese	Baked beans
Baked beans	Mashed potatoes
Broccoli with almonds	Broccoli
Peanut-butter-stuffed celery	Peanut-butter-stuffed celery
Custard	Cake
3. LACKING VARIETY IN COLOR	
Omelet	Vegetable scallops with tartar
Sweet potatoes	sauce
Squash	Sweet potatoes
Carrot salad	Asparagus
Sponge cake	Coleslaw
	Raspberry sherbet
4. LACKING VARIETY IN TEXTURE	
Cheese soufflé	Cheese soufflé
Mashed potatoes	Oven-browned potatoes
Cauliflower	Green beans
Molded salad	Lettuce wedges
Vanilla pudding	Vanilla pudding
5. TOO RICH, AND REPETITIOUS OF CHEESE	
Nut loaf	Gluten loaf with tomato sauce
Potatoes au gratin	Baked potatoes
Fried eggplant	Fried eggplant
Frozen fruit salad (with mayonnaise, whipped cream)	Tossed green salad
Cheesecake	Cheesecake

Adapted from Bogert, Briggs, and Calloway, *Nutrition and Physical Fitness,* 8th ed., p. 492.

day's chili on a future day for patties. Checking the menu in advance ensures having items when needed. Even out peak loads for crowded days by preparing food ahead.

Planning for Time and Abilities and Use of Energy

Making the menu coincide with time and abilities is important in menu planning. If you know that you have only a short time available at mealtime, utilize convenience foods or prepare major items the day before. Often you can dovetail jobs, such as baking dessert for tomorrow while you do today's dishes. An automatic oven set in advance to produce the fragrant finished product as the family arrives makes a pleasant homecoming.

Consider also equipment size and availability. If you have only one oven, it limits the number of items you can bake at one time. On the other hand, bake several dishes at a time rather than heat the oven just to bake potatoes. As a rule, a slight variation in temperature indicated on the recipe will not greatly affect the end product. The lowest temperature recommended for baking any of the items generally does quite well for the several dishes prepared for the meal. If one dish requires a longer baking time, start it baking before you put the second item in the oven. Electric frying pans and microwave ovens may be real energy- and time-savers. A rack in a microwave oven may make possible the preparation of a whole meal in the oven at one time. We do need to conserve on scarce and costly heat energy. This is very important in planning. But appliances that you do not use regularly only clutter available space.

Time, experience, for physical strength may limit the abilities of the individual who will prepare the meals, and prepared or partially prepared foods may become a necessity. In a limited situation, you may be able to make a specialty requiring extra time if you can prepare the remainder of the meal quickly and easily.

Food Budget Facts

The budget may require some manipulating of the jigsaw, but planning ahead assists the juggling act. Limited money for food need not make meals dull, uninteresting, or inadequate. Neither does a liberal budget guarantee good nutrition or even pleasing and satisfying meals. Incorporate the economical principles of purchasing discussed in the chapter "Food Puzzle Applied." Then, supported by a shopping list compiled from the menus, you may avoid the pitfalls of impulse buying. Attractive food displays frequently form the financial downfall of the buyer without a plan. How much of the available income to spend for food is not easy to answer. The figure varies according to the family's size and set of values. Regardless of the amount spent, fulfilling the requirements of the Four Food Groups is the first prerequisite. Since this simple four-piece puzzle offers unlimited variety, altering the choices within each group can greatly reduce food costs.

Advertising alerts the food buyer to reduced prices on items in large supply or in season, and the wise shopper experiences substantial savings by taking advantage of advertised sales. Descriptive terms in newspaper advertisements, as well as food labels, indicate quality, size, and kind of pack. Price alone does not indicate a good food buy. In taking advantage of a special, do not allow impulse buying to lure you. Purchasing a large quantity of something the family dislikes or that will spoil quickly does not constitute a savings. Shopping when hungry may tempt the shopper to buy high-cost extras, such as potato chips, just because of an attractive display. Menus may be changed to take advantage of bargains and seasonal items. Almost everyone enjoys corn on the cob, tomatoes, and fresh peaches daily when they are in season. Buying an item just because it is reduced in price does not save money if you do not incorporate it into the menu.

All management requires flexibility. Circumstances necessitate adaptation, but planning gives security and a base from which to make the necessary changes. The homemaker who plans attractive menus from foods the family likes is well on the way to a successful food puzzle picture, thus supplying good nutrition within her budget of time, energy, and money.

Meals for Special Occasions

A hostess need not feel that planning and preparing meals for guests suggests an overwhelming task. Once you master the practice of planning menus on paper, you can quickly write the menu for company meals. Why not tuck in the recipe box several special menus for immediate reference?

The special menus may include a buffet menu, a picnic menu, seasonal menus for planned dinner guests, and a menu or two you can quickly put together with foods from an emergency shelf.

When writing or choosing a menu for guests, decide first the type of service you will use. For a large group, a buffet is practical and pretty, and the wise hostess selects easily prepared recipes. Use a casserole, salad, and dessert that you can prepare in the morning or the day before. Make the cold beverage in advance and allow it to chill. Just before the meal, prepare the relishes while the casserole heats and the vegetables cook. If you make the relishes earlier, cover them well and refrigerate. Spread the breads and pour the beverage just before you arrange the hot food on the buffet table. To generate smiles, serve a light dessert as a final touch.

At a picnic, the hostess can enter into the fun more fully than in other types of entertaining. It also can serve as practice for more formal occasions. When planning the picnic menu, choose foods that require little preparation at the picnic site, or that keep well when prepared ahead. Remember during the picnic season the advice to be found in the chapter "Poison in the Pot."

Most families and guests look with approval at the picnic table when something new or unusual appears. New and appealing recipes from magazines, newspapers, and cookbooks provide fresh ideas.

For a spontaneous summer picnic, the children will enjoy sandwiches as the main dish, since they carry no lunches when outdoor meals are in vogue. A mixture of canned and fresh seasonal fruit (in disposable cups), relishes, beverage, and dessert will round out a carefree meal.

Meals including several families and eaten potluck style require planning to ensure a well-balanced menu. The hostess, keeping in mind the specialties of her friends, may tactfully suggest items for each one to bring. Even families on a limited budget and working women with little food preparation time can enjoy potluck meals.

For the more formal occasion, dinner guests anticipate an appointment when they know that a relaxed hostess awaits their arrival. The old saying "Practice makes perfect" applies in meal service too. The unsure hostess can practice serving a formal menu to the family before serving guests. It is easier to invite just two or three guests to dinner at first.

Getting ready well in advance, as for the buffet, the hostess will not give guests the impression of having overworked in preparing for them. By using a menu that includes two or three items that can bake together, she avoids last-minute crises.

Set the table the final stages of meal preparation. When you invite guests for dinner after church, or for supper after a lecture or concert, set the table before leaving home. Then you can welcome your guests and spend but little time for last-minute touches and placing the hot food.

What about unexpected guests, however? Every hostess should realize that the meal is only a small part of entertaining. A longtime friend coming without notice will go away remembering a wonderful

AN-9

visit. When a stranger comes to church and you invite him for dinner, he remembers a friendly church. When a new family moves into town and is invited for dinner, they begin to feel they belong. Unexpected guests will soon forget the food served but will long remember the hospitality extended.

Many hostesses keep an emergency shelf containing all the items required for menus planned for unexpected guests. These items might include ingredients for a quick, casual stroganoff, canned baked beans, or canned vegetables if you have no room in the freezer for any emergency items. Especially for weekends, store in the refrigerator lettuce, cabbage, and tomatoes for a fresh salad. Dessert can be as simple as instant pudding topped with canned fruit and served with a cracker or cookie. Cold water will do very nicely for a beverage if one is needed and you have nothing else on hand.

Do not avoid inviting guests to the home because you feel unable to please them. Although there are many rules for meal planning and proper service, today's society allows a hostess great flexibility in her own home. Advance planning and preparation frees a hostess to enjoy the company of her friends while serving fancy meals on special occasions, and entertaining them becomes a pleasure.

A backward glance at the table before calling the family or guests should give real satisfaction to the home artist who has planned and executed her plan carefully.

Section IV

On Your Guard
132/Poison in the Pot
137/Current Quackery
142/Food Fads and Facts

Chapter 13

POISON IN THE POT

Some attractively prepared and served foods may be unsafe to eat. Invisible toxic agents that give no warning of their presence by flavor, odor, or appearance cause food poisoning. Hours, or even days, after eating a toxic food, sickness or death may strike. Food poisoning occurs one of three ways: (1) from toxic substances occurring naturally in food, (2) from bacteria in food, or (3) from toxins produced by bacteria living in food.

Food Toxins

The toxic substances occurring naturally in plants and animals receive comparatively little attention today. In past ages, man discovered by trial and error which "foods" caused sickness and death. Such items cannot be purchased in grocery stores. Owing to constant surveillance by the Food and Drug Administration, this country's food supply is wholesome and reliable. Foods that do not meet government standards are quickly removed from the market. The *FDA Papers* publish monthly the reports of such recalled items and of the Food and Drug Administration's continuing search for safer and improved foods.

Although the foods purchased are reliable, some toxic plants grow in every area of the country and may be obtained through channels other than the grocery store. Anyone involved with the food preparation needs to know naturally occurring toxins.

Many varieties of mushrooms are poisonous—some so deadly that merely handling one and then touching the fingers to the mouth can transfer a fatal amount of toxin. Since several of the edible mushrooms have poisonous "look-alikes," no one but an expert with adequate experience should decide which are edible. Consumers not qualified to select wild mushrooms should use only those grown commercially. Several types of mold and fungi related to mushrooms may grow on otherwise edible foods and cause poisoning. Never eat dry grains, nuts, corn, legumes, or any food that shows evidence of mold.

Certain raw foods contain toxic substances that heating inactivates. Common examples are soybeans and lima beans. These legumes are entirely safe after cooking. The fava bean, whether cooked or raw, has frequently been reported to cause poisoning in individuals sensitized to it.

Solanine is a toxic agent in sprouting potatoes, or those that have turned green from exposure to light. Cut away green areas on potatoes, for they contain solanine. Rhubarb leaves can cause illness because of a concentration of oxalic acid, whereas the young stems can be eaten without harm.

Some persons fear "can poisoning" from commercially canned foods refrigerated in their open cans. The can will not cause poisoning; however, it may impart a metallic flavor to the food after opening, caused by the reaction of food acids and air on the metal can. Tomatoes and tomato juice commonly develop a metallic flavor from opened cans, which, although not poisonous, certainly does not add to palatability.

Occasionally foods are poisoned by substances that get into them by mistake. Store separately and clearly label all cleaning supplies, insecticides, and any other nonfood items kept in the kitchen. Always store such nonfoods out of the reach of youngsters.

Somewhat obliquely related to food poisoning is the question occasionally raised concerning the radioactive contamination of food. With increased use of radioactive materials, the government agencies who protect food supplies continually monitor the level of such materials in food. Milk is frequently used as an index, for cows forage over large areas and could ingest quantities of radioactive compounds. The fact that milk is used as a reference food, and is occasionally associated with radioactivity in reports, does not make it any less safe than other foods subject to radioactive contamination.

Bacterial Food Toxins

The more common form of food poisoning results from bacterial contamination of food. Bacteria, like people, require various nutrients for their growth; thus the more nutritious combinations provide excellent media for bacterial growth. The living bacteria themselves or the toxins produced by bacteria may cause food poisoning.

Various bacteria of the genera *Salmonella* and *Streptococcus* cause poisoning by infecting the host. *Staphylococcus* organisms produce toxins that cause poisoning. Within two to forty-eight hours after ingestion of these bacteria or their toxins, the symptoms of poisoning may occur: nausea, vomiting, abdominal cramps, and diarrhea. Death from such poisoning is rare; complete recovery usually takes one to three days. Severe cases may require hospitalization in which fluids and electrolytes (mineral salts) lost by vomiting and diarrhea are replaced intravenously to prevent dehydration and mineral imbalance.

For poisoning by these bacteria to occur, four conditions must exist:

1. *Food providing an excellent nutrient media for rapid bacterial growth.*

Foods upon which these bacteria vegetate are those rich in protein and carbohydrates, often in combinations such as cold meat salad, potato salad, cream puddings and pies, custards, stuffed eggs, and cream puffs. Since acid ingredients slow bacterial growth, add lemon juice to potato salad, egg salad, and protein sandwich fillings.

2. *Inoculation of the bacteria into the food.*

This occurs easily in many ways. The food handler may contaminate the food by unwashed hands that have touched pimples or come in contact with intestinal excreta, or hands that have even a small infection on them; by droplets from talking or coughing over food when the handler has an infected throat; or by tasting from a stirring spoon or licking the fingers. (Poisoning by staphylococci is most commonly introduced in these ways.) Never use hands for mixing foods, especially those foods that you do not heat before serving. It is also the food handler who likely contaminates foods with salmonellae. Only rarely and under "dirty" conditions does the disease originate from rodent, fly, or cockroach contact with the food, or from diseased meat. If a cow or hen is infected by salmonellae, pasteurization of the milk and at least soft boiling of the egg destroy all these organisms.

3. *Room temperature.*

With nutrient material available, bacteria multiply very rapidly at room temperature. Refrigeration temperatures delay their growth, but only after the entire mass of food has cooled. For prompt cooling, thinly spread foods that readily support bacterial growth. Freezing stops bacterial multiplication but does not kill the organisms. When frozen foods thaw, the bacteria again become active, and precautions must be taken to prevent their growth.

4. *Sufficient time for bacterial growth.*

Under the proper conditions, bacteria can multiply sufficiently within two to three hours to cause poisoning. Every food handler should assume that foods like those mentioned in item No. 1 have been inoculated, and either serve them immediately, before bacteria can multiply, or refrigerate or freeze the food, to prevent multiplication. Never allow these foods to remain at room temperature.

Botulism is another type of food poisoning caused by toxins produced by living bacteria. This poisoning is dealt with individually because it is unique in several ways.

Clostridium botulinum spores are common and not harmful. Only when they remain alive in airtight containers and are not destroyed by heat do they produce a deadly toxin. One taste from a jar infected with growing botulinal organisms could supply a fatal dose of the toxin, which attacks the nervous system rather than the gastrointestinal tract. Fatigue, visual disturbances, and muscular paralysis lead to death from respiratory muscle failure. Whereas the other types of bacterial food poisoning rarely kill, botulism kills approximately 65 percent of those infected.

Toxins of *C. botulinum* are not formed in a distinctly acid media, which includes most fruits. The most common source of this poisoning is home-canned vegetables (green beans, corn, beets, spinach, asparagus) and home-canned meats or sea foods. *C. botulinum* spores are present in the soil in many areas and thus may remain on subacid foods when canned. The spores withstand boiling temperatures, then begin to grow inside the sealed jar. When the jar is later opened, no physical change in the food appears, yet one taste of the food may result in death.

To make home-canned foods safe, follow these precautions:

1. Pressure-can subacid foods (vegetables, meats, and meat analogs) according to pressure and timetables published by reliable sources (Ball Brothers Company, Incorporated, Muncie, Indiana; Kerr Field Services Department, Sand Springs, Oklahoma; United States Department of Agriculture, Home and Garden Bulletins). Only pressure canning heats the food sufficiently above boiling temperature to kill the spores that could later produce the toxin.

2. Boil home-canned subacid vegetables for ten minutes before tasting or serving. Sufficient boiling renders toxin-poisoned foods safe. Even so, nonpressure canning of subacid foods is not recommended. One thoughtless taste could kill.

Freezing or commercial canning renders subacid foods safe.

It is imperative for safety that all food handlers are educated to the existence of the unseen micoorganism world. A classic example to the contrary is the uninformed housewife who, in the days before really cold refrigeration, placed yesterday's potato salad on the table while telling her friend of vague digestive tract upsets and sickness that had troubled her family frequently that summer. The friend, eyeing the potato salad, suggested maybe their trouble was food poisoning. The housewife replied in a huff, "I don't put poison in my food!"

To be sure prepared foods are safe, remember the following points: Promptly serve or quickly refrigerate all high-nutrient foods that are handled or are in close contact with people and are served unheated. In refrigerating such food, spread it three inches or less in depth and leave uncovered until thoroughly chilled. High-risk foods such as potato salad, egg salad, and meat sandwiches should not be served at picnics or in lunches unless the people furnishing these foods understand how to handle them. Thoroughly chill such foods immediately after preparation and then hold them not more than two hours out of refrigeration. Never bring unused foods conducive to the growth of bacteria home from picnics. Pressure-can all subacid foods, then, when opened, boil thoroughly before tasting.

Individuals involved in food handling must know that what they prepare is completely safe. If there is the slightest question as to the safety of a food, adopt the motto "When in doubt, throw it out!"

Chapter 14

CURRENT QUACKERY

Today's sophisticated consumer smiles when he reads accounts of uninformed old-timers who fell prey to the nutritional-quackery vendors of the "good ole days." They hawked mystical snake oils, wolf milk, or cure-all tonics under the flicker of torches and to the beat of drums, promising relief of ills and revitalization of life. After finishing the entertaining article, this same intelligent American will likely include costly vitamin pills or food supplements with his dinner. This educated individual is convinced that supplements or specially grown foods prevent subclinical deficiencies, which he feels sure will result from eating inadequate foods grown on depleted soil, and which processing further devitalizes.

This sophisticated, intelligent consumer is only today's version of yesterday's snake-oil buyer, now fallen prey to a laboratory-coated charlatan who dispenses quack diets and fake supplements that promise a shortcut to health. By a clever blending of science with superstition and a smattering of pseudoscientific terms, the propagandist can easily persuade and present apparently plausible theories that promise much.

Individuals likely to fall into faddism can usually be classed in one of four categories: (1) those who adopt new ideas and diet systems from fashion rather than concerning themselves with the facts behind the ideas, (2) those who worry about their state of health and feel there must be some way to make their current good health better, (3) those with real illnesses who find it easier to believe bizarre claims of a quack than ethical medical advice, or (4) neurotic individuals who derive psychological reassurance from following an unusual diet plan. Eating uncommon or even disliked foods comforts these individuals.

The food faddism racket is a multi-billion-dollar business. Every report indicates that food quackery is continuing to rise despite the efforts of regulatory agencies and educational programs. Many faddish notions are relatively harmless healthwise. They merely relieve one of his money and are ridiculous when viewed through the scientific eye. But when promoters claim cures for diseases or symptoms not caused by a dietary deficiency at all, or when one follows the fad cure instead of getting proper medical attention, tragic results can follow.

Many fad diets restrict their followers to a few rather unusual or exotic foods. The human body needs the variety of nutrients that a variety of common foods best supplies. Often the faddist keeps in relatively good health by "fad hopping." Fad diets can grow very monotonous, which luckily drives the faddist to try new systems. A grapefruit diet one week, yogurt and molasses the next, followed by a raw carrot and hard-boiled egg jag may ultimately furnish the needed nutrients to prevent nutritional deficiencies, although it is far from an ideal dietary pattern.

As a result of mass communication devices and educational accomplishments, the American consumer is very health conscious. *Low-calorie foods, polyunsaturated fats, trace minerals, minimum daily requirements*—all are terms used in everyday conversation. The consumer is constantly made aware of important nutritional advancements, but he rarely has the specialized knowledge necessary to distinguish between nutritional sense and nonsense.

The advice of self-styled nutritionists, overzealous salesmen, best-selling so-called nutrition books, or the more subtle advertising gimmicks need not bewilder. To put himself in control, the consumer needs to become an informed skeptic—informed on factual guidelines, and skeptical of any person or product that does not measure up to ethical standards.

Evaluating the Source

Believe it if the information comes from—
> The American Dietetic Association.
> The American Institute of Nutrition.
> The American Society for Clinical Nutrition.
> The U.S. Department of Agriculture and the Food and Drug Administration.
> State departments of health.
> University nutrition departments.
> Nutrition sections of the following scientific groups:
>> The American Medical Association.
>> The American Public Health Association.
>> The American Home Economics Association.
> Individuals who have an academically recognized degree in

nutrition or dietetics, such as the registered dietitian.
Beware if the advice is from:

Someone with something to sell.

That a large portion of the American public will accept
doorbell "doctors" or mailed circulars as the last word on
nutrition is amazing. Question the authority of anyone with
a product to sell. (Do not confuse this point with fully
qualified persons employed by an ethical food or equipment
company who give correct information about nutrition or the
product's use.)

One posing under an authoritative title (doctor, professor,
nutritionist, biochemist) but who lacks credentials necessary to support such a title.

Quickly discredit the "authority" if he claims that accepted
scientific organizations persecute him. No amount of piety
can replace true competence. The intelligent individual
must watch out for quotations from reputable nutrition
authorities that someone takes out of context or warps to
suit his own ends.

A person who is a professional in another field but not in
nutrition.

Educated individuals may be authorities in their area, but
possessing an advanced degree in another area does not
make one a nutrition authority.

A well-meaning but uninformed friend.

Personal testimonies are a most believable promotional
gimmick. They may cleverly sell a product. Your friend may
sincerely believe what he says, but the fact remains that all
the sincerity in the world does not make a false idea true.

Popular books on nutrition.

Many of them contain some good information mixed with
misinformation. Frequently they contain medically and
nutritionally unsound advice. Such books are dangerous and
unsuitable for reference.

Evaluating the Information

Do not believe it if:

It guarantees exuberant health or everlasting youth.

It blames all ill health entirely on poor nutrition.

It says you cannot get proper nourishment from foods because
of depleted soil or overprocessing.

It recommends any one "miracle food" or "loaded" formula.

A reducing program allows you to eat anything you desire.
It offers a cure for a condition that ethical medical science thus far has been unable to remedy.
It is straight misinformation, such as:
"Grape juice constitutes a good source of vitamin B_{12}."
"The composition of avocado and milk is similar. Use avocado in the place of milk."
"Honey is a food; refined sugar is a poison."
"Arrowroot flour has a high calcium content."

Outright false statements are frequently the most difficult to recognize unless the doubter is trained in nutrition or has a reliable source of information. False statements are commonly made in regard to the composition of foods. Every interested individual should have a reliable food composition booklet. Then when a self-styled nutritionist or a new cookbook says that honey is a good source of minerals or that almonds can be made into a milk substitute, the composition reference will show these claims to be completely erroneous. Two excellent sources for reliable compositions of foods are the U.S. Department of Agriculture Home and Garden Bulletin No. 72, with foods listed in common serving portions, and the U.S. Department of Agriculture Handbook No. 456.

When evaluating diet systems for reducing, gaining, or a myriad of other reasons, the most reliable guide is: Do they measure up to the Four Food Groups without warping the picture? Overemphasis or exclusion of any one group signals a nutritional imbalance. A nonfortified beverage made from soybeans, belonging to the protein group, cannot replace foods in the milk group. You cannot ignore the cereal group just because you wish to eat only an abundance of fruit. All foods have been assigned their position in one of the Four Food Groups according to their nutrient content. Wishing a food into another group will not change its nutritive contribution to the diet.

The most reliable guide to remember when confronted with a "miraculous" potion is: No one food or supplement is the key to good health. The human body needs the correct balance of nutrients, and common foods best furnish these. The swindler may claim that fatigue or nervousness or any number of vague aches and pains are the result of something lacking in the diet and that his special dietary food or capsule will absolutely cure them. "True, $39.99 a month, but when the family's *health* is at stake, money should be of no concern," he cajoles. By gulping loaded pills, potions, or entire diets, without a physician's direction, the gullible are likely to incur imbalances that could never occur if they ate common foods as outlined by the Four

Food Groups. For instance, a continuous overdose of especially vitamin A or D can lead to hypervitaminosis—a serious toxic condition, especially if children or expectant mothers are the victims.

The following chapter lists some of the more commonly believed fallacies, along with explanations of the nutritional facts.

Chapter 15

FOOD FADS AND FACTS

Many faddish ideas spring from nutritional facts warped to suit someone's personal motives. Just the right amount of truth blended with the erroneous, along with a slight play on the emotions, and the charlatan has built a very convincing story and probably a lucrative business. The following are examples of commonly encountered fallacies, with explanations of the facts.

● Soils are so impoverished that our foods lack nutrients.

Neither poor soil nor rich soil affects the composition of plants and their seeds or fruits. The quality of the soil definitely affects the crop yield, but not its nutritional quality. Plants need certain elements for growth and reproduction and simply will not grow if the required elements are not available. Different strains of the same food plant may vary somewhat in nutrient content because of genetic variations. For example, different varieties of oranges develop slightly different amounts of vitamin C. Because of this fact, food composition listing from different sources will show some variations. New strains of food plants are constantly developed, such as corn higher in lysine and tomatoes with more vitamin C. The genetic code, not soil fertility, determines the composition of a plant.

Historically, iodine deficiency has resulted from exclusively eating foods grown where the soil lacks iodine. Today deficiencies in micronutrients are almost unheard of in industrialized countries because modern storage and transportation bring foods from many regions into local areas. Sufficient iodine is easily obtained by using iodized salt.

● Commercial liquid or dry formulas are most effective in weight reduction.

Any diet plan of six hundred calories daily or less will cause a dramatic weight loss. The first liquid protein diets were of the poorest, nonsustaining quality proteins. These formulas were followed by better quality protein sources. However, when calories (energy) are sparse, protein is used to meet the body's energy needs.

When strictly followed, medical complication can range from dizziness, nausea, and weakness, to collapse and even death. No one should follow such a restricted diet plan without continuously monitored supervision by a physician. The weight loss is rarely permanent because the individual may not have learned to alter his eating plan.

Weight, usually gained slowly, is most safely lost slowly with an appropriate exercise program combined with a controlled calorie intake from common foods that meet all nutrient requirements. Only food can supply both known and unknown nutrients in safe balance.

• Monoglycerides and diglycerides come from animal sources and can be added to fats labeled as "pure vegetable."

Monoglycerides and diglycerides may be derived from either animal or vegetable sources. Chemically speaking, they are related to fats and may be considered partially digested fats. Enzymes in the intestinal tract break each fat molecule (Figure 1, below) by a stepwise process, first into a diglyceride (Figure 2) and one fatty acid, then into a monoglyceride (Figure 3) and two fatty acids, and finally into an alcohol (glycerol) and three fatty acids (Figure 4), which the body absorbs.

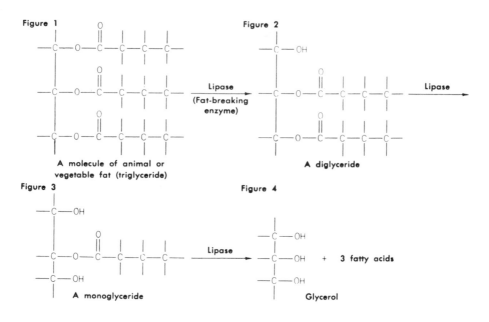

Figure 1

A molecule of animal or vegetable fat (triglyceride)

Lipase (Fat-breaking enzyme)

Figure 2

A diglyceride

Lipase

Figure 3

A monoglyceride

Lipase

Figure 4

Glycerol   +   3 fatty acids

The chemist can "digest" animal or vegetable fats in the laboratory to produce monoglycerides and diglycerides. The source of these pure chemical entities is usually stated on the label. They are added in extremely small amounts (usually around one tenth of 1 percent) to margarine and butter to make them more spreadable.

● Pesticides poison our foods. Chemical food additives are dangerous.

When foods are grown without protection, healthy bugs and a decreased crop result. Without some means of control, food crop pests would cause incalculable damage every year, resulting in a scarcity of food and increased costs. So pesticides are important to us.

But do pesticides poison our foods? No, because crop pesticides have a very limited active life. Those permitted for use become inactive within hours or a few days after their application. Spraying schedules and harvest times are controlled.

Food additives have received a great deal of attention from food manufacturers and consumers. Those who have no knowledge of chemistry tend to become emotional at the thought of chemicals in their food. Yet every item in our world is a chemical or a mixture of chemicals: flowers, the Mackinac Bridge, food, cells in the human body.

Certain additives benefit, such as vitamins and minerals added in carefully regulated amounts. Additives such as emulsifiers and stabilizers facilitate processing. Spoilage retardants increase keeping ability and provide food the consumer expects at prices he can afford. In many ways food additives are responsible for the superior selection and quality of the foods we enjoy. Without them it would be impossible to feed the masses.

Before a food processor receives permission to use an additive, it must be proved safe by biological testing. Food additives are under constant study by the Federal Government, private agencies, and educational centers, and after passing government standards for safety, study on the additives' long-term effects continues. If such research shows extended use or cumulative amounts to be harmful, the additive is removed from the approved list.

Dr. Harvey W. Wiley, a founder of the present Food and Drug Administration, which is directly responsible for consumer protection, made a guiding statement in 1867: "We are carefully to preserve that life which the Author of nature has given us, for it was no idle gift."

● Natural organically grown foods are superior to chemically fertilized foods.

Food crops need certain nutrients for growth just as do human beings. The plant cares not whether the elements it draws from the soil came from decomposing organic matter or from a sack of "chemical" fertilizer. All nutrients are chemical compounds. Nitrogen is nitrogen, iron is iron, sodium is sodium—its source does not matter, only whether it is present or lacking in the soil. If certain nutrients are scarce, the crop yield will be small but nutritionally equal to lush crops grown in rich soil. Large-scale crop nutrient needs can best be met by commercially prepared fertilizers. Without current-day knowledge of soils and the use of all types of fertilizers, this nation's food crop yield would greatly diminish, and food prices would skyrocket.

• Cooking or commercial processing destroys the nutritive value of foods.

Many a food cultist promotes a diet totally composed of foods in their natural state. Although some raw fruits and vegetables are desirable, the human digestive system is not constructed to handle great quantities of raw materials as the grazing animal's digestive system can. The body more easily and completely digests certain foods when properly cooked; thus we derive greater nutritive value from them. Modern food-processing methods quick-freeze or can fruits and vegetables at their peak nutritional value.

Some consider white flour, refined cereals, or any number of other processed foods devoid of nutritional value. This is simply not true. While it is always preferable to obtain foods in as natural a form as possible, one cannot say that processed foods are worthless. Instant dry potatoes, powdered milk, et cetera, have a significant nutritional contribution to make. White flour and refined cereals have had the major nutrients replaced that were lost through extensive processing. Thiamine, riboflavin, niacin, and iron are replaced to correspond approximately with the food's original nutritional level.

• One must eat raw foods for their enzymes.

Cooking temperatures inactivate enzymes—complex specks of nonliving proteinaceous matter. Plants and animals produce hundreds of different enzymes for their very specialized needs. Plant enzymes help bring about maturity and ripening. The enzymes essential to human life function in digestion, absorption, metabolism of foods, and building and repair of cells. Living cells secrete each enzyme to perform its very specific function. Enzymes produced within our own bodies cannot be interchanged. Digestive enzymes secreted into the digestive tract could never replace the enzymes needed to handle foodstuff once it is in the bloodstream. Our bodies

AN-10

cannot adopt the enzymes in raw plant foods. The best to be said of plant enzymes is that they are harmless. The body digests the eaten enzymes and may utilize the microscopic bit of protein. Every normal living organism makes all its own enzymes or hosts the necessary bacteria that make enzymes to fit all its own needs.

● Natural vitamins are better than synthetic vitamins. Every one should take vitamins.

A vitamin is a chemical compound with a specific structure. Hand a laboratory-produced "synthetic" vitamin sample and an extracted "natural" vitamin sample to an analytic biochemist, and he would not find any difference between the two. Structure and function identify a vitamin; its origin makes no difference.

Not everyone should take vitamins. Concentrated vitamin preparations should be considered medicine and taken only under a physician's direction. Self-medication may be only a costly waste or may lead to a serious toxic condition. The body cannot store water-soluble vitamins (vitamin C and most of the B vitamins) for the simple reason that they dissolve in water, and excesses are excreted. Taking an overabundance of these vitamins wastes money. However, the body stores the fat-soluble vitamins (especially vitamins A and D), which may lead to the toxic condition hypervitaminosis. Hypervitaminosis is frequently a conundrum. Symptoms of the condition may resemble the deficiency symptoms of the vitamin involved. Both too little and too much vitamin A or D may result in poor growth, nausea, diarrhea, itching skin, or headache. If you follow the Four Food Groups, you will never ingest toxic amounts of the vitamins and minerals naturally present in foods.

● Eating hard fats will raise the cholesterol level, and this may cause heart attacks.

Consumption of hard animal fats and/or hard (hydrogenated, saturated) vegetable fats does tend to increase the blood cholesterol level. An elevated blood cholesterol level may be one factor leading to coronary heart disease, and moderate changes in food selection can reduce the amount of cholesterol in the bloodstream. First, the average American should cut down on fat intake; then, replace hard fats with small amounts of seed oils or products made from these nonhydrogenated oils (high in polyunsaturates).

Cholesterol is a normal, useful body constituent originating from synthesis within the body and from foods. Conforming to a very strict cholesterol-free diet may cause considerable inconvenience to the individual, besides those near and dear, and may result in little or no change in blood cholesterol levels, because of the body's ability to make cholesterol.

ABOUT NUTRITION

An elevated cholesterol level is not the only cause of heart attack. High blood pressure, overweight, too little physical activity, cigarette smoking, tensions and stresses, eating largely of simple carbohydrates (all sugars and honey), diabetes, and heredity are all risk factors. An individual can reduce or eliminate these risk factors, with the exception of heredity, if he so chooses.

A physical examination by a physician should include a blood analysis that shows not only the cholesterol level but also gives a profile of all blood fats. If a person is at risk, the diet and lifestyle can be modified to improve the blood fat profile.

• Honey is high in minerals and will not cause tooth decay. Refined sugar is a poison; raw sugar is a food.

A brief table clearly compares the various forms of sugar:

	Cal.	Pro. gm.	Fat gm.	Ca. mg.	Phos. mg.	B₁ mg.	B₂ mg.	Niacin mg.
Whole milk, 1 cup	160	9	9	288	227	.08	.42	0.1
Avocado (½), 123 grams	160	2	14	12	52	.13	.24	2.0
Almonds, ¼ cup	212	6	19	83	46	.08	.33	1.2

Honey is a poor source of minerals, especially when one considers the number of calories it contains. As for not causing tooth decay, honey's mixture of sucrose, fructose, and glucose does not differ from any other sugar in that respect. Any sugar in the mouth encourages bacterial growth, which in turn produces decay-causing substances.

White sugar (sucrose) is refined from cane and beets by man. Honey is also a refined product. The bee drinks nectar, concentrating and changing it from its original form before placing it in the comb. The only real choices between these two forms of sugar are (1) whether the individual prefers either man or bees to have concentrated this high-calorie food, and (2) the taste difference. One advantage of honey might be its greater flavor and sweetness, thus tiring the taste buds more quickly than would white sugar, so that one might eat less.

Refined sugar is raw sugar with the molasses removed; brown sugar is refined sugar with a controlled amount of the molasses returned to the sugar. Whether the sweetness comes in granular or syrupy form, or in dark or light color, it is still sugar—a simple carbohydrate and a concentrated calorie source one should limit in the diet.

Although blackstrap molasses does contain considerable amounts of minerals, it cannot be considered a common mineral source. The average individual consumes very little blackstrap molasses in a year's time, and appreciable amounts irritate the gastrointestinal tract.

• Avocado "milk" furnishes the same nutrients as cow's milk and can be used in its place. Almond "milk" can be made for children.

The only substance legally termed *milk* is the secretion of the mammary gland. Milk is a superb blend of nutrients manufactured to meet the very exacting needs of the growing mammal. Avocado or almonds or any other fruit or nut made into "milk" can never exactly replace milk. In terms of protein alone, no single plant protein is completely balanced in the essential amino acids necessary for growth. A correct mixture of different vegetable proteins can furnish all the essential amino acids, but when nuts, seeds, or avocado makes up the majority of the mixture, the fat (and calorie) content becomes prohibitive. Milk makes an especially important contribution to the body's calcium and phosphorus needs. The body best absorbs and utilizes these two minerals when they are eaten in approximately a one-to-one ratio, which milk closely provides. Milk is definitely superior to fruit or nut preparations during the months of life when physical and mental development largely depend upon a formula food.

1 Tablespoon	Calories	Calcium	Iron mg.
White sugar	45	0	trace
Honey	65	1	0.1
Corn syrup	60	9	0.8
Brown sugar	50	12	0.5
Molasses, light	50	33	0.9
Molasses, blackstrap	45	137	3.2

• Homemade or "health" baking powders are better than commercial preparations. Alum and lime are harmful substances sometimes included in commercial baking powder.

Baking powder combines an edible acid and alkali with a drying ingredient that helps prevent moisture from accumulating, which would cause the two to react and loose carbon dioxide prematurely. The acid and alkali portions must be very precisely weighed and combined so that each reacts totally with the other (stoichiometrically balanced), leaving little or no alkaline and, no acid residue. Commercial baking powders can be more carefully produced with precision equipment so that they are stoichiometrically balanced and leave only a neutral residue. Home measuring of baking powder components lacks precision and leaves true balancing of ingredients to chance. An excess of alkali (soda) leaves an alkaline residue that destroys B vitamins and irritates the digestive tract.

The so-called "health" baking powder, available under several common brand names, is a calcium phosphate product. The body can use the neutral calcium phosphate salt left in the food after baking.

Alum is not harmful. Many of our foods contain aluminum salts. The idea that aluminum injures began somewhere in the dusty past during trade wars between competitive baking powder companies and competitive cooking utensil companies. The fact that this idea is totally unfounded has not dulled its popularity over the years. Lime is another name for calcium oxide—calcium is essential to life.

• Milk and sugar ferment in the stomach to produce alcohol.

If milk and sugar produced alcohol in the stomach, few would patronize the beer and wine industries. Any individual wishing to go on an alcoholic binge could do so just by eating these very available and inexpensive foods. Likewise, anyone not wanting to wash his problems away in alcohol would become drunk from merely eating food. A few extremely rare individuals have hosted abnormal gastrointestinal bacteria that could produce alcohol from food, and they remained in a drunken stupor most of the time until medical science could eradicate the unusual microorganisms.

Sugar is classed chemically as an alcohol, as are many of our foodstuffs. These food alcohols and alcohols resulting from normal digestion do not cause inebriation.

Fermentation means the decomposition of a substance into simpler substances. Sugar does "ferment" during the normal process of digestion, for it is broken down into simpler sugars. Fermentation could also be an acidic fermentation, which in this case does not result in the formation of alcohol, but this type of fermentation can cause discomfort and "indigestion." This can be caused by eating large quantities of milk and sugar.

Possibly the fact that sugar is classed as an alcohol, or a misconception of the word *fermentation*, has led to the erroneous idea that sugar ferments in the stomach to produce inebriating alcohol.

● Alcohol is formed as yeast dough rises.

True. Fallacy enters when persons become concerned that some lingers when the bread is eaten warm.

For optimum growth yeast requires sugar, moisture, and a warm temperature. The tiny yeast plants utilize sugar if it is present in the dough, or they can produce an enzyme capable of converting some of the starch of flour into sugar. As the yeast multiplies, it produces carbon dioxide gas, causing the dough to rise. Some ethyl alcohol also results. This alcohol is very volatile, and the heat of the oven rapidly drives it off. No alcohol remains in baked bread.

● Megadoses of vitamins and minerals improve health.

When a vitamin enters the body, it travels to a cell that needs it and attaches to a protein made in the cell. Only then is the vitamin able to perform its specific nutritional duties. The proteins that combine with vitamins have their needs filled when the person eats vitamins at the recommended daily levels. Any extra vitamin coming into the cell cannot possibly serve its vitamin function, because the cell needs no more and has no more specific protein receptors available.

All vitamins are chemicals. Megadose excesses can function only as chemicals and not as vitamins. For instance, megadoses of vitamin C may raise the uric acid level and may precipitate gout in people so predisposed. Also, vitamin C in great excess may impair the function of vitamin B_{12}. A patient with diabetes, determining how much insulin he should take by checking his urine, may get into serious trouble from megadoses of vitamin C, which causes one urine sugar tester, Tes-Tape, to be false-negative, and a different tester, Clinitest, to be false-positive. Another problem is that the strong reducing action of megadoses of vitamin C causes false-negative readings for blood-in-the-stool tests, which could result in a failure to diagnose intestinal disorders, including carcinoma of the colon.

Scientific advancements in crop propagation, storage, and transportation have blessed our country with a great variety of nutritious foods. The individual can meet his nutritive needs by eating readily available inexpensive foods. If a person happens to like the flavor of yogurt, wheat germ, carrot juice, and sprouted alfalfa and has the extra time and money to supply himself with these less common foods, he should be allowed to eat them in moderation without being classed as a faddist. But when an individual eats these rather unusual foods to the exclusion of more common ones or when he thinks the unusual foods nutritionally superior, he has become a faddist. Faddish beliefs are especially hurtful when they lead one to buy costly specialty foods or home-sized processing equipment out of a limited budget and in place of good food. Common foods abundantly furnish all the nutrients needed. The reward for eating these common foods according to the Four Food Groups is excellent nutritional health. Correct nutrition provides the best insurance in all stages of life.

FOOD AND NUTRITION BOARD, NATIONAL ACADEMY OF SCIENCES—NATIONAL RESEARCH COUNCIL RECOMMENDED DAILY DIETARY ALLOWANCES.[a] Revised 1980

Designed for the maintenance of good nutrition of practically all healthy people in the U.S.A.

	Age (years)	Weight (kg.)	(lb.)	Height (cm.)	(in.)	Protein (g.)	Fat-soluble Vitamins Vita-min A (µg. RE)[b]	Vita-min D (µg.)[c]	vita-min E mg. α-TE)[d]	Water-solu Vita-min C (mg.)	Th mi (m
Infants	0.0 − 0.5	6	13	60	24	kg x 2.2	420	10	3	35	0
	0.5 − 1.0	9	20	71	28	kg x 2.0	400	10	4	35	0
Children	1 − 3	13	29	90	35	23	400	10	5	45	0.
	4 − 6	20	44	112	44	30	500	10	6	45	0.
	7 − 10	28	62	132	52	34	700	10	7	45	1
Males	11 − 14	45	99	157	62	45	1000	10	8	50	1
	15 − 18	66	145	176	69	56	1000	10	10	60	1
	19 − 22	70	154	177	70	56	1000	7.5	10	60	1
	23 − 50	70	154	178	70	56	1000	5	10	60	1
	51 +	70	154	178	70	56	1000	5	10	60	1
Females	11 − 14	46	101	157	62	46	800	10	8	50	1
	15 − 18	55	120	163	64	46	800	10	8	60	1
	19 − 22	55	120	163	64	44	800	7.5	8	60	1
	23 − 50	55	120	163	64	44	800	5	8	60	1
	51 +	55	120	163	64	44	800	5	8	60	1
Pregnant						+30	+200	+5	+2	+20	+0
Lactating						+20	+400	+5	+3	+40	+0

[a] The allowances are intended to provide for individual variations among most normal persons as they live in the United States under usual environmental stresses. Diets should be based on a variety of common foods in order to provide other nutrients for which human requirements have been less well defined.

[b] Retinol equivalents. One retinol equivalent = 1 µg. retinol or 6 µg. β carotene.

[c] As cholecalciferol. Ten µg. cholecalciferol = 400 IU of vitamin D.

[d] A-tocopherol equivalents. One mg. d-α tocopherol = 1 α-TE.

[e] ONE (niacin equivalent) is equal to 1 mg. of niacin or 60 mg. of dietary tryptophan.

[f] The folacin allowances refer to dietary sources as determined by *Lactobacillus casei* assay after treatment with enzymes (conjugases) to

mins				Minerals					
Niacin (mg. NE)[e]	Vita-min B6 (mg.)	Fola-cin[f] (µg.)	Vitamin B12 (µg.)	Cal-cium (mg.)	Phos-phorus (mg.)	Mag-nesium (mg.)	Iron (mg.)	Zinc (mg.)	Iodine (µg.)
6	0.3	30	0.5[g]	360	240	50	10	3	40
8	0.6	45	1.5	540	360	70	15	5	50
9	0.9	100	2.0	800	800	150	15	10	70
11	1.3	200	2.5	800	800	200	10	10	90
16	1.6	300	3.0	800	800	250	10	10	120
18	1.8	400	3.0	1200	1200	350	18	15	150
18	2.0	400	3.0	1200	1200	400	18	15	150
19	2.2	400	3.0	800	800	350	10	15	150
18	2.2	400	3.0	800	800	350	10	15	150
16	2.2	400	3.0	800	800	350	10	15	150
15	1.8	400	3.0	1200	1200	300	18	15	150
14	2.0	400	3.0	1200	1200	300	18	15	150
14	2.0	400	3.0	800	800	300	18	15	150
13	2.0	400	3.0	800	800	300	18	15	150
13	2.0	400	3.0	800	800	300	10	15	150
+ 2	+0.6	+400	+1.0	+ 400	+ 400	+150	h	+ 5	+ 25
+ 5	+0.5	+100	+1.0	+ 400	+ 400	+150	h	+10	+ 50

make polyglutamyl forms of the vitamin available to the test organism.

[g] The recommended dietary allowance for vitamin B12 in infants is based on average concentration of the vitamin in human milk. The allowances after weaning are based on energy intake (as recommended by the American Academy of Pediatrics) and consideration of other factors, such as intestinal absorption.

[h] The increased requirement during pregnancy cannot be met by the iron content of habitual American diets or by the existing iron stores of many women; therefore the use of 30-60 mg. of supplemental iron is recommended. Iron needs during lactation are not substantially different from those of nonpregnant women, but continued supplementation of the mother for 2-3 months after parturition is advisable in order to replenish stores depleted by pregnancy.

U.S. DIETARY GOALS (Revised)*

GOALS

1. To avoid overweight, consume only as much energy (calories) as is expended; if overweight, decrease energy intake and increase energy expenditure.
2. Increase the consumption of complex carbohydrates and "naturally occurring" sugars from about 28 percent of energy intake to about 48 percent of energy intake.
3. Reduce the consumption of refined and processed sugars by about 45 percent to account for about 10 percent of total energy intake.
4. Reduce overall fat consumption from approximately 40 percent to about 30 percent of energy intake.
5. Reduce saturated fat consumption to account for about 10 percent of total energy intake; and balance that with polyunsaturated and monounsaturated fats, which should account for about 10 percent of energy intake each.
6. Reduce cholesterol consumption to about 300 milligrams a day.
7. Limit the intake of sodium by reducing the intake of salt to about 5 grams a day.

SUGGESTED CHANGES IN FOOD SELECTION AND PREPARATION

1. Increase consumption of fruits and vegetables and whole grains.
2. Decrease consumption of refined and other processed sugars and foods high in such sugars.
3. Decrease consumption of foods high in total fat, and partially replace saturated fats, whether obtained from animal or vegetable sources, with polyunsaturated fats.
4. Decrease consumption of animal fat, and choose meats, poultry, and fish which will reduce saturated fat intake.
5. Except for young children, substitute low-fat milk for whole milk, and low-fat dairy products for high-fat dairy products.
6. Decrease consumption of butterfat, eggs, and other high-cholesterol sources. Some consideration should be given to easing the cholesterol goal for premenopausal women, young children, and the elderly in order to obtain the nutritional benefits of eggs in the diet.
7. Decrease consumption of salt and foods high in salt content.

---

* From Senate Nutrition Comittee, *Dietary Goals of the United States,* revised, January, 1978, Superintendent of Documents, U.S. Government Printing Office, Washington, D.C. 20402, $2.30.

Basic References for *About Nutrition*

American Dietetic Association. *Vegetarian Position Paper.* Chicago: American Dietetic Association, 1980.

Food and Nutrition Board, National Research Council, National Academy of Sciences. *Toward Healthful Diets.* Washington, D.C.: National Academy Press, 1980.

Food and Nutrition Board, National Research Council. *Recommended Dietary Allowance.* 9th ed. Washington, D.C.: National Academy of Sciences, 1980.

Select Committee on Nutrition and Human Needs, U.S. Senate. *Eating in America: Dietary Goals for the United States,* 2d ed. Cambridge, Mass.: MIT Press, 1977. Also available from the Government Printing Office, Washington, D.C., under the title *Dietary Goals for the United States,* 1978.

United States Department of Agriculture. *Nutritive Value of American Foods, in Common Units,* by Catherine F. Adams. Agriculture Handbook No. 456. Superintendent of Documents, U.S. Government Printing Office, Washington, D.C. 20402, 1975.

The U.S. Department of Agriculture and the Surgeon General, U.S. Department of Health and Human Services. *Dietary Guidelines for Americans.* Washington, D.C.: U.S. Government Printing Office, 1980.

White, Ellen G. *Counsels on Diet and Foods.* Washington, D.C.: Review and Herald Pub. Assn., 1946.

General Reference Books

Alford, Betty B., and Margaret L. Bogle. *Nutrition During the Life Cycle.* Englewood Cliffs, N.J.: Prentice-Hall, 1982.

Bennion, Marion. *Introductory Foods.* 7th ed. New York: Macmillan Pub. Co., 1980.

Briggs, George M., and Doris H. Calloway. *Nutrition and Physical Fitness.* 11th ed. New York: Holt, Rinehart and Winston, 1984.

Brody, Jane. *Jane Brody's Nutrition Book.* New York: Bantam Books, 1982.

Calloway, Doris Howes, and Kathleen O. Carpenter. *Nutrition and Health.* Philadelphia: Saunders College Pub., 1981.

Carey, Ruth L., Irma B. Vyhmeister, and Jennie Stagg Hudson. *Commonsense Nutrition.* Mountain View, Calif.: Pacific Press Pub. Assn., 1971.

Charley, Helen. *Food Science.* 2d ed. New York: John Wiley and Sons, 1982.

Christian, Janet L. and Janet L. Greger. *Nutrition for Living.* Menlo Park, Calif.: Benjamin/Cummings Pub. Co., 1985.

Endres, Jeannette B., and Robert E. Rockwell. *Food, Nutrition, and the Young Child.* St. Louis: C. V. Mosby Co., 1980.

Fleck, Henrietta C. *Introduction to Nutrition.* 4th ed. New York: Macmillan Pub. Co., 1981.

Fonosch, Gail G., and Elaine Friedkin Kvitka. *Meal Management.* San Francisco: Canfield Press, 1978.

Fretz, Sada. *Going Vegetarian: A Guide for Teen-agers* (recipe section). New York: William Morrow and Co., 1982.

Hafen, Brent Q. *Nutrition, Food, and Weight Control.* Expanded ed. Boston: Allyn and Bacon, 1981.

Hamilton, Eva May, and Eleanor N. Whitney. *Nutrition: Concepts and Controversies.* 2d ed. St. Paul: West Pub. Co., 1982.

Heslin, Jo-Ann, Annette Natow, and Barbara Raven. *No-Nonsense Nutrition for Your Baby's First Year.* Boston: CBI Pub. Co., 1978.

Kart, Cary S., and Seamus P. Metress. *Nutrition, the Aged, and Society.* Englewood Cliffs, N.J.: Prentice-Hall, 1984.

Kinder, Faye, and Nancy R. Green. *Meal Management.* 5th ed. New York: Macmillan Pub. Co., 1978.

Lowenberg, Miriam E., et al. *Food and Man.* 2d ed. New York: John Wiley and Sons, 1974.

Mayer, Jean. *A Diet for Living.* New York: David McKay Co., 1975.

McGill, Marion, and Orrea F. Pye. *The No-Nonsense Guide to Food and Nutrition.* New York: Butterick Pub., 1978.

McWilliams, Margaret. *Fundamentals of Meal Management.* Fullerton, Calif.: Plycon Press, 1978.

Moore, Shirley T., and Mary P. Byers. *A Vegetarian Diet.* Santa Barbara, Calif.: Woodbridge Press Pub. Co., 1978.

Notelovitz, Morris, and Marsha Ware. *Stand Tall! The Informed Woman's Guide to Preventing Osteoporosis.* New York: Bantam Books, 1985.

"Nutrition Misinformation and Food Faddism." *Nutrition Reviews* (Special Supplement), July, 1974.

Pipes, Peggy L. *Nutrition in Infancy and Childhood.* 3d ed. St. Louis: C. V. Mosby Co., 1984.

Seventh-day Adventist Dietetic Association. *Diet Manual, Including a Vegetarian Meal Plan.* Margaret Kemmerer Heath, ed., 6th ed. Box 75, Loma Linda, Calif. 92354, 1982.

Stare, Fredrick J., and Margaret McWilliams. *Nutrition for Good Health.* Fullerton Calif.: Plycon Press, 1974.

White, Phillip L., and Nancy Selvey. *Let's Talk About Food.* Acton, Mass.: Publishing Sciences Group, 1974.

Whitney, Eleanor N., and Eva May N. Hamilton. *Understanding Nutrition.* 3d ed. St. Paul: West Pub. Co., 1984.

Williams, Sue Rodwell. *Mowry's Basic Nutrition and Diet Therapy.* 7th ed. St. Louis: Mosby College Pub., 1984.

Worthington-Roberts, Bonnie Sue, et al. *Nutrition in Pregnancy and Lactation.* 3d ed. St. Louis: C. V. Mosby Co., 1985.

Cookbooks

Calkins, Fern, U. D. Register, and Lydia Sonnenberg. *It's Your World Vegetarian Cookbook.* 2d ed. Washington, D.C.: Review and Herald Pub. Assn., 1981.

Cottrell, Edyth Young. *The Oats, Peas, Beans & Barley Cookbook.* Santa Barbara, Calif.: Woodbridge Press, 1974.

Goldbeck, Nikki, and David Goldbeck. *American Wholefoods Cuisine.* New York: New American Library, 1983.

Nelson, Ethel R. *Century 21 Cookbook.* Rev. ed. Eusey Press, 1974.

Vollmer, Marion W. *Food for Your Health and Efficiency.* 2d ed. Hagerstown, Md.: Review and Herald Pub. Assn., 1983.

For Use in Cooking Schools

Fagal, Sylvia M. *Nutrition Helps.* Rev. ed. Seventh-day Adventist Dietetic Assn., 1985.

Marsh, Alice G. *Supplement for Demonstration Techniques.* Berrien Springs, Mich.: Department of Home Economics, Andrews University, 1985.

Register, Helen H. *Food Preparations and Nutrition Education.* Abundant Living Health Series, vol. 4. Loma Linda, Calif.: School of Health, Loma Linda University.

Specific Studies

American Dietetic Association. Position paper on the vegetarian approach to eating. *Journal of the American Dietetic Association,* 77(1980): 61.

American Heart Association (and its State affiliations). Request recent literature. 44 East 23d St., New York, N.Y. 10010.

American Institute for Cancer Research. *Planning Meals That Lower Cancer Risk: A Reference Guide.* P.O. Box 76216, Washington, D.C. 20013, 1984. Designed for health professionals.

Heaney, R. P., et al. "Calcium Nutrition and Bone Health in the Elderly." *American Journal of Clinical Nutrition,* 36 supp. (1982): 986.

Linkswiler, H. M., et al. "Protein-induced Hypercalcariuria." *Federation Proceedings,* 40(1981): 2429.

Marsh, Alice G., et al. "Bone Mineral Mass in Adult Lacto-ovo-vegetarian Males." *American Journal of Clinical Nutrition,* vol. 37 (March, 1983).

———, et al. "Cortical Bone Density of Adult Lacto-ovo-vegetarian Women." *Journal of the American Dietetic Association,* vol. 76 (February, 1980).

National Research Council. *Diet, Nutrition, and Cancer.* Bethesda, Md.: National Cancer Institute, 1982.

Phillips, Roland. *Adventist Health Studies.* Loma Linda, Calif.: Loma Linda University.

Spencer, H. H., et al. "Studies in Calcium Requirement in Man." Reprint of original data and review. *Clinical Orthopedics,* in press (1984).

Journals of Lay and Professional Interest

Nutrition Today. Cortez F. Enloe, Jr., M.D., ed. 428 E. Preston Street, Baltimore, Md. 21202.

Vibrant Life. Ralph Blodgett, ed. 55 West Oak Ridge Drive, Hagerstown, Md. 21740.

INDEX

Abilities in meal planning, 127
Acids and alkalies, effect of on ingredients, 119
Additives, chemical, 143-145
Alcohol, 149, 150; in yeast dough, 150; not recommended, 94
Almond "milk," 148
Altitude, effect on cookery, 118, 119
American Cancer Society, 94
American Heart Association, 94, 95; recommendations for low fat in diet, 95
Amino acids, 45; complete and incomplete, 46; essential, 46; high and low biological value, 46
Anabolism, 29
Analogs, meat, 109
Anorexia nervosa, 87
Antioxidants, 40
Ariboflavinosis, relation to riboflavin, 63
Ascorbic acid, 26, 66, 67
Atherosclerosis, 41
Avocado "milk," 148
B vitamins, 61-64
Babies, feeding, 70-72
Bacterial food toxins, 133-136
Baking powder, use, 108; "health," 149; alum in, 149; trade wars, 149
Beriberi, relation to thiamine, 63
Beverages, 113
Bone mineral loss, 96; fracture region, 96, 97
Botulism, Clostridium botulinum, 135, 136
Bran, cereal, 36, 37
Brassica vegetables, 93, 94
Bread crumbs, measuring, 115
Breadmaking, 106-108; formula for, 108
Breakfasts, 123-125
Breast feeding, 70
Budget, food, 127
Buffet foods, 128, 129
Bulimia, 87
Caffeine, 95, 96
Calcium, 26, 51, 52; bone decalcification, 52; common food sources, 55, 90, 91; greens as a source of, 51; heartbeat, dependent on, 51; loss of, 96; milk as a source of, 51; normal clotting of blood, 51
Cancer, 93, 94
Canning, home, precautions for, 135
Carbohydrates, 34; digestion of, 35
Carotenes, 59

Catabolism, 29
Cellulose, 35
Cereals, cooked and prepared, 105; enrichment of, 36, 105; nutrient loss by washing, 106
Children, feeding, infant, 70-72; toddler, 72-74; preschool, 74-76; school-age, 76-78; teens, 78-81
Chocolate and cocoa, 113
Cholesterol, 40, 43, 95; in hard fats, 146, 147
Chromium, 54
"Clean plate," 75
Clostridium botulinum, 135
Cookbooks, use of, 115, 116
Cooking, "waterless," nutrient loss in, 102; nutrient value of food in, 145
Coronary heart disease, 94, 95, 146
Cruciferous (brassica) vegetables, 93, 94
Dental health, 90, 91; sugar-caused decay, 147
Desserts, 112, 113
Detergent foods, 91
Dextrins, 35
Dextrose, 34
Dietary Goals of the United States, 39
Diets, crash, 84; weight loss, 83, 84
Digestion of food, 31, 35, 48
Diglycerides, 143, 144
Disaccharides, 35
"Dowager's hump," 96
Eggs, cholesterol in yolks of, 43; cooking of, 110
Enrichment of cereals and flour, 36, 105
Energy metabolism, 34, 48, 49
Enzymes, raw food, 145, 146
Essential substances (nutrients), 38
Evaluating information, 138-140
Faddism, food, 137, 138; evaluation of, 138-141
Faddist, faddish, 150, 151
False-negative and false-positive urine tests, 150
Fats, 37-45; digestion of, 45, 143; hard, hydrogenated, 38, 39; monounsaturated, 38, 95; polyunsaturated, 38, 39; P/S ratio, 39-44; unsaturated, 38, 95
FDA Papers, 132
Fiber, 36, 37, 105
Fermentation, 149, 150
Flour, enriched, 36, 105; whole-grain, 36
Fluoridation, water, 90, 91
Fluorine, 50, 53, 54

Food and Drug Administration, 132, 144
Food and Nutrition Board, 152, 153
Food fads, 137-151; facts, 137-151
Food groups, additions, 23-26; applied, 16-26, 100; calculating content of, 27; evaluating the diet by, 140
Food likes and dislikes, 125
Food poisoning, 132-136; high-risk, 134; toxins, 135
Food preparation, environmental factors affect, 117, 118
Food puzzle, applied, 100-114; fruit and vegetable group, 100-104; bread and cereal group, 104-108; protein group, 108-111; milk group, 111-114
Formulas, liquid and dry, 142
Four Food Groups, 16-29
Freezing food, 135
Fructose, 34, 92
Frying, 118
Galactose, 34
Generic foods, 101
Glucose, 34, 92
Gluten, preparation of, 109, 110
Glycerides, mono- and di-, 143
Glycogen, 35
Gout, 65, 150
"Grazing," 76
Growth, rapid, 26
Health risks, reducing, 93
Heart disease, coronary, 94, 95; risk factors, 41
Heat conduction, 117
Hemicellulose, 36
Honey, 23, 147
Hydrogenation of fats, 38
Hypervitaminosis, 64; of A and D, 141
Impacting foods, 91
Infant feeding, 70-72
Infarct, 40
Information, evaluating nutritional, 138-141
Iodine, 50, 53, 142
Iron, 26, 52, 53; menstrual loss, 52, 53; overload, 26; sources, 56
Lactation, 23
Lactose, 35, 92
Laxatives, habit-forming, 37, 105
Leftovers, 125
Legumes, cooking, 109
Levulose, 34
Lignin, 36
Lime, 149
Linoleic acid, 38, 41-43
Lipids, blood, 43
Lipoproteins, 40; HDL and LDL, 40
Lunches, pack-it, 122
Maltose, 35

Meal planning, aesthetics in, 125; breakfasts, 120; buffet, 128, 129; common errors in, 126; guest, 129, 130; menus, 121-126; milk in, 123; a pattern for, 124; picnic, 129; protein in, 123; special occasions, 128-130; suppers, 121; timing, 127
Measuring ingredients, 116
Megavitamin therapy, 64, 65
Menu planning, see Meal planning
Metabolism, 29; energy, 48, 49, 50
Microminerals, 54
Milk, essential nutrients in, for dental health, 91
"Milk," nut and vegetable, 148
Milk, reconstituting, 116
Milk and sugar, 149
Milk group, 111-113
Minerals, 50-56, 105; megadoses, 150
Misinformation, food, 137-141
Molasses, blackstrap, 147
Monoglycerides and diglycerides, 143, 144; from fats, 45
Monosaccharides, 34, 35
National Academy of Sciences, 93, 152, 153
National Cancer Institute, on *Diet, Nutrition, and Cancer,* 93, 94
National Research Council, 48, 152, 153
Niacin, 63, 64, 66, 67
Nibbling, 85
Nutrients, functions, 30; loss of in fruits and vegetables, 118
Nutrition, lifetime, 70
Nutritional information, evaluation of, 138-140
Oil, seed, unhardened, 42, 43
Organically grown foods, 144, 145
Osteoporosis, 52, 96
Overnutrition, 13
Overweight, 83-89
Oxidation, 34
Pectin, 36
Pellagra, relation to niacin, 63, 64
Pesticides, 143
Picnic foods, 129
Phosphorus, 90, 91
"Planned-overs," 125
Plaque, dental, 90
Poisons, food, 132-136
Polysaccharides, 35
Pregnancy, eating plan for, 22, 23
Preschooler, feeding, 74-76
Processed foods, 105
Processing food, 36, 145
Protein, food sources 47, 90, 91; high biological value, 26, 46
Protein group, 108-111

Proteins, common food sources, 47; cooking of, 108-111; digestion of, 46; purchasing of, 109
Proteins and the amino acids, 45-48
P/S ratio, 39, 44
Quackery, current, 137-141
Radioactive contamination, 133
Raw foods only, 145
Recommended Daily Dietary Allowances, 24, 152, 153
Riboflavin, 63, 66, 67
Risk factors in heart disease, 41, 83, 84, 147
Saccharide units, 34
Salads and dressings, 103, 104
Salmonella, 133-136
Salt, iodized, 142
School-age children, basic meal plan for, 21
School-age feeding, 76-78
Scurvy, 62, 65
Self-feeding during the second year, 73, 74
Seventh-day Adventists and alcohol, 93, 94
Snack foods, 76
Soda, neutralizing, 107, 108
Soil, impoverished, 142
Sorbitol, 92
Special occasions, meals for, 128-130
Spiritual facets, supported by nutrition, 13
Staphylococcus, 133
Starches, 35
Streptococci, cariogenic, 92; toxins, 133-136
Sucrose, 34, 35, 92
Sugar, fructose, 34; galactose, 35; glucose, 34; lactose, 34, 35; maltose, 34, 35; mineral content of, 147, 148; raw, 147, 148
Teens, 78-81; eating patterns for, 22
Teeth, nutrition and care of, 90-92
Temperature in cooking, 118
"Terrible twos," 73
Thiamin, 63, 66, 67
Timing in meal planning, 127
Toddler, 72-74
Toxins, food, 132; bacteria producing, 133; by contamination, 136; fava beans contain, to sensitized persons, 133; in green potatoes, 133; in moldy grains, 132, 133; in mushrooms (certain varieties), 132; in raw soybeans and lima beans, 133; in rhubarb leaves, 133
Triglycerides, 40
Tryptophan, 26, 64

Undernutrition, 13
Underweight, 87-88
Uric acid, 150
U.S. Dietary Goals, 37, 39, 43
Vegetable protein cookery, 116
Vegetables, cancer risk-reducing, 93, 94; green and yellow, 17, 123; soda not recommended in cooking, 102; strong-flavored, 102
Vitamin A, deficiency symptoms, 59, 60; fortification of milk, 111; from green and yellow vegetables, 26, 58-60, 123; hypervitaminosis, 141, 146; megadoses, 65; reduces cancer risk, 66, 67, 94; tooth formation, 90, 91
Vitamin B-complex, 62-65; effect of acids and alkalies on, 119, 149; effect of soda on, 102; in whole grains, 66, 67, 105
Vitamin B^6, megadoses, 65
Vitamin B^{12}, 64; deficiency leading to nerve degeneration, 64; in red cell formation, 64; present in animal foods, 64; with excess of vitamin C, 150
Vitamin C, best source, 62; at breakfast, 123; destroyed by air, 117; destroyed by alkalies, 119; excess, 65; in Four Food Groups, 26; in megadoses, causes false negative urine test, 150; in megadoses, effect on vitamin B$_{12}$, 150; in tooth formation, 91; increased by genetic manipulation of plants, 142; not stored in body, 146; protects against scurvy, 62; requirement easily met, 62; role in reducing cancer risk, 94; role of, 62, 66, 67
Vitamin D, 61; hypervitaminosis, 141, 146; in tooth formation, 90, 91; milk fortified with, 111; toxicity, 65
Vitamin E, 60; effect of megadoses, 65
Vitamin K, 60, 61
Vitamins, best sources of, 58, 66, 67; destroyed by excess soda, 149
Water, 54, 113, 114; fluoridation of, 90; in cooking, 117, 118
Weaning infants, 72
Weight, reducing, 83-89, 95; underweight, 87, 142, 143; use of Four Food Groups, 84, 85
Weights and measures in food preparation, 115, 116
White, Ellen G., regarding nuts, 110
Women, postmenopausal, 26, 51, 52
Women, premenopausal, 52
Yeast, 106, 150
Yogurt, recipe, 112
Zinc, 54